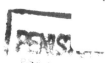

Award-winning writer, television broadcaster and author of numerous bestsellers, **Leslie Kenton** is described by the press as the 'guru of health and fitness' and 'the most original voice in health'. A shining example of energy and commitment, she is highly respected for her thorough reporting. Leslie was born in California, and is the daughter of jazz musician Stan Kenton. After leaving Stanford University she journeyed to Europe in her early twenties, settling first in Paris, then in Britain where she has since remained. She has raised four children on her own by working as a television broadcaster, novelist, writer and teacher on health and for fourteen years was health and beauty editor at *Harpers & Queen*.

Leslie's writing on mainstream health is internationally known and has appeared in *Vogue*, the *Sunday Times*, *Cosmopolitan*, and the *Daily Mail*. She is the author of many other health books including: *The New Raw Energy* – co-authored with her daughter Susannah – *The New Biogenic Diet*, *The New Joy of Beauty*, *The New Ageless Ageing*, *Cellulite Revolution*, *10 Day Clean-Up Plan*, *Endless Energy*, *Nature's Child*, *Lean Revolution*, *10 Day De-Stress Plan* and *Passage to Power*. She turned to fiction with *Ludwig* – her first novel. Former consultant to a medical corporation in the USA and to the Open University's Centre of Continuing Education, Leslie's writing has won several awards including the PPA 'Technical Writer of the Year'. Her work was honoured by her being asked to deliver the McCarrison Lecture at the Royal Society of Medicine. In recent years she has become increasingly concerned not only with the process of enhancing individual health but also with re-establishing bonds with the earth as a part of helping to heal the planet.

Also by Leslie Kenton

THE JOY OF BEAUTY
ULTRAHEALTH
RAW ENERGY (with Susannah Kenton)
RAW ENERGY RECIPES (with Susannah Kenton)
AGELESS AGEING
THE BIOGENIC DIET
10 DAY CLEAN-UP PLAN
CELLULITE REVOLUTION
ENDLESS ENERGY (with Susannah Kenton)
NATURE'S CHILD
LEAN REVOLUTION
10 DAY DE-STRESS PLAN
THE NEW JOY OF BEAUTY
THE NEW ULTRAHEALTH
THE NEW AGELESS AGEING
THE NEW BIOGENIC DIET
THE NEW RAW ENERGY (with Susannah Kenton)
PASSAGE TO POWER
RAW ENERGY FOOD COMBINING DIET
JUICE HIGH (with Russell Cronin)
TEN STEPS TO ENERGY
REJUVENATE NOW
THE RAW ENERGY BIBLE
TEN STEPS TO A NEW YOU

QUICK FIX SERIES
Boost Energy
Look Great
Sleep Deep
Get Fit
Lose Fat
Beat Stress

Fiction
LUDWIG (a spiritual thriller)

Ten Steps to a **Natural Menopause**

Leslie Kenton

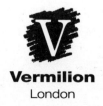

Vermilion
London

1 3 5 7 9 10 8 6 4 2

Text copyright © Leslie Kenton 1999

The right of Leslie Kenton to be identified as the author
of this book has been asserted by her in accordance
with the Copyright, Designs and Patents Act, 1988.

First published in the United Kingdom in 1999 by Vermilion
an imprint of Ebury Press
Random House
20 Vauxhall Bridge Road
London SW1V 2SA

Random House Australia (Pty) Limited
20 Alfred Street, Milsons Point, Sydney,
New South Wales 2061, Australia

Random House New Zealand Limited
18 Poland Road, Glenfield,
Auckland 10, New Zealand

Random House South Africa (Pty) Limited
PO BOX 337, Bergvlei, South Africa

Random House Canada
1265 Aerowood Drive, Mississauga
Ontario L4W 1B9, Canada

Random House UK Limited Reg. No. 954009

A CIP catalogue record for this book is available
from the British Library

ISBN: 0 09 182546 6

Printed and bound at Cox and Wyman, Reading, Berks

Contents

Author's Note

The content of this book is intended for informational purposes only. I am only a reporter. None of the suggestions or information are meant to be prescriptive. Any attempt to treat a medical condition should always be under the direction of a competent physician – preferably one knowledgeable about nutrition and natural methods of healing. Neither the publishers nor the author can accept responsibility for injuries or illness arising out of a failure by a reader to take medical advice.

I want to make clear that I have no commercial interest in any product, treatment or organisation mentioned in this book. However, I have long sought to learn more about whatever can help us to live at a high level of energy, intelligence and creativity, for it is my belief that the more each one of us is able to re-establish harmony within ourselves and with our environment, the better equipped we shall be to wrestle with the challenges now facing our planet.

Step One
Go Free

Power, energy and freedom are the rewards of a natural menopause. This is a book about how to make them part of your life. It is not about how to cope with 'the horrors of the change'. Instead it reveals that the transformation menopause brings to a woman's life is a journey towards individual freedom. It is a voyage of discovery which, step by step, explores the misconceptions surrounding menopause, investigates the implications of environmental pollutants and hormone 'treatments', and uncovers the role diet and lifestyle can play in protecting women from menopausal misery. It also gathers together diverse information about simple yet effective action a woman can take to improve her physical health and appearance as well as to maximise her energy and enhance the quality of her life, whatever her age.

Changing Perspective

Nobody ever prepares you for menopause. Nobody tells you that if you are going to have hot flushes or emotional instability they are likely to be far worse before you stop menstruating than afterwards. Nor does anybody explain that waking regularly at two or three in the morning and lying in bed filled with sadness or fear or anger is likely to be not a sign of illness, but a messenger announcing that menopause is near. Because we are told so little, few women in our culture are prepared for the intensity of emotion – both anguish and joy – that can accompany the end of the child-bearing years, nor do they know what to do with it. Despite my knowledge about health I was totally unprepared for 'the change'. I had no idea of the freedom that is available to us on the other side of it. Not the freedom advertisers would have us believe comes with a pair of Levi 501's or using the right tampon or sanitary towel so we can 'have fun' at any time of the month. It is a freedom of body and soul which enables each woman to live out the truth of who she is and to experience unfettered her full enjoyment of life. The first step towards a natural menopause is to claim your right to freedom. But to do this you need to make a shift in the way you think about menopause itself.

The radical and fundamental changes which take place in a woman's life around the time of menopause are not signs of decay or pathology, but part of an exciting adventure. This is a time to regenerate and rejuvenate our bodies, to unearth parts of our personality that have been hidden beneath the responsibilities of the child-bearing years, a time to discover that our creativity is no longer bound to our obligation as a member of the human race to propagate the species. Now that the child-bearing years have ended, menopause brings the freedom to surrender to passionate love-making without fear of pregnancy, or to refuse sex altogether if we choose. It brings freedom from the emotional ups and downs that often accompany menstruation, as well as freedom to feel radiantly fit and well. You no longer need to be bound to your role as mother or servant, wife or lover. Anthropologist Margaret Mead claimed that passing through menopause brought a woman 'post-menopausal zest'.

What is Menopause?

The horror stories we hear about menopause today are so far removed from what was once, and should still be, a wonderfully positive experience that women are beginning to ask themselves just what is going on. Is menopause a cosmic joke, an aberration of evolution? Did Nature screw up when she made us this way? Are we meant to be over the hill at fifty? If we don't take HRT right away are we going to end up as crumpled old bags in ten years? Or, even worse, dead after having broken both hips falling down the stairs? These are the questions menopausal women I have worked with in Britain, North America, Australia, New Zealand and South Africa have been asking me for years. They reflect women's fears, and the exhortations to which they are now subjected. It is not easy to know what to make of it all. To enjoy the benefits of a natural menopause we need to become well informed. Each of us needs to become familiar with what lies behind the various symptoms commonly associated with menopause in the West, and find out how relatively easy it can be to counter them, often without having to resort to serious medical intervention of any kind.

Strictly speaking, just as the word 'menarche' means a woman's first menstrual period, 'menopause' means the last period she will ever have. *Meno* comes from the Greek meaning 'month', and pause from *pausis*, meaning 'halt'. In common usage, however, when most people speak of menopause they are talking about the whole of the period a woman goes through – often for years before and after her last menstruation – during which the production of reproductive hormones (oestrogens and progesterone) slow down, her periods may become irregular and she begins to experience other bodily signs of change, ranging from sudden fluctuations in temperature to alterations in sleep patterns. This total transition from the child-bearing to the past-child-bearing years is properly known as *the climacteric*. And, because each woman is a biochemical and physiological individual, it can last from a few months to as long as ten or fifteen years. The climacteric is usually divided into three parts: peri-menopause, the time when hormonal shifts have already begun but a woman is still menstruating; menopause, the time at which the last period occurs; and post-menopause. The end of a woman's reproductive life seldom coincides with the time of her last period. It can come before or afterwards. This is the main reason why it is important to continue to use some sort of contraception for the first year to eighteen months after your last period if you don't want another child.

This all sounds very natural and simple. So what has gone wrong?

Fear of Change

On a physical level, the proliferation of poisonous chemicals in our environment and the widespread use of chemically grown convenience foods have dangerously eroded our freedom to be healthy, so much so that we now experience a Pandora's box of ailments – from infertility and PMS to cancers of the womb and breasts – with a frequency and intensity unprecedented in history. Meanwhile, driven by a desire to exploit the largest commercial market in the world, drug manufacturers spend a fortune each year in an attempt to convince governments, doctors and the public that using their products for contraception and to treat problems which arise as menopause approaches is the only choice available to women. Faced with the prospect of a menopause increasingly portrayed as dangerous to body and mind, as an event which can turn an attractive woman into a confused old hag, women can become frightened into complying, sometimes to their long-term detriment. Our fears of menopause need to be seen for the paper dragons they are.

To some women, even a hint that menopause may be on its way is confirmation that they are 'past it', or that 'it's all downhill from here,' and they look for a way to halt it. At some point in mid-life every woman in our society comes to feel the sadness and frustration which arise because our society links physical ageing to the loss of sexual attractiveness and self-esteem. So when menopause arrives it can seem an unwelcome visitor, a symbol of one's depreciating sexual worth. Women who have long been at home may find that home and family have ceased to hold the fascination they once had; they may no longer seem good sources from which to draw a sense of personal identity. On the other hand, women who have had a career may come to feel that although they may have achieved the success they once longed for, something fundamental is missing. They ask themselves if life is not passing them by.

Quick Fix?

A woman nearing menopause is particularly vulnerable to any suggestion about how life is going to change. If she is told that menopause is a deficiency disease or an inevitable source of struggle, pain and grief that will undermine her sexual attractiveness and push her over the hill, she is likely to face her future burdened with these notions. Once a woman, even unconsciously, swallows the negative stereotypes that our culture has created about older women, she opens herself up to the idea that she needs 'treatment' – much as she can be convinced that she needed a designer suit, a three-piece suite, a new lover, or a BMW to make her life work. The only problem is that such things rarely deliver the gifts they promise.

As any marketing folk worth their salt know full well, the easiest way to sell anything to a woman is to convince her that she is inadequate and in desperate need of whatever they offer. This is exactly what has happened with hormone replacement therapy (HRT). Information on menopause is not readily available to women, apart from those cheerful little booklets on the subject from doctors' surgeries which are little more than thinly disguised vehicles for the sale of HRT. Even the best-written articles in women's magazines and in newspapers tend to follow closely the medical-industrial 'catechism'. In recent decades, backed by major pharmaceutical money, an obsession with HRT has developed. As a result, in the past thirty years very little objective research into other aspects of menopause and the hormonal changes associated with it has been carried out. By far the most revealing investigations into the nature of menopause have been carried out not by medical researchers but by anthropologists, psychologists, sociologists and epidemiologists. As a result, despite all the books and articles published on the subject and all the leaflets that are handed out, surprisingly little objective medical information is yet available about the menopausal woman. The people who know most about natural menopause are the women who have passed through it themselves.

Fearful Symptoms

When you examine the scientific studies that have been conducted into menopause you realise that many of the so-called symptoms of menopause have nothing in particular to do with it. They are instead symptoms of ageing, or imbalances that have developed out of lifestyles that do not give real support to the proper functioning of mind and body. Or they are symptoms of frustration at the very deepest levels that arise when a woman is trying to live everybody else's life rather than her own. Such 'menopausal' symptoms can include aches and pains, fatigue, digestive disturbances and anxiety – all of which develop when a woman's metabolic processes are not functioning as they should be. They may be the result of years of eating convenience foods short of essential minerals and trace elements and full of junk fats. They can also develop when a woman has been wrestling with the long-term stress of a marriage that isn't working or a career that demands everything of her yet brings her little satisfaction in return. Around the time of mid-life all of these things get thrown together and wrongly labelled 'the symptoms of menopause'. Treating them with tranquillisers or hormone drugs is simply papering over the cracks.

Spiritual Interface

Like the moon's waxing and waning, a woman is a cyclic creature. This is a result of the almost infinitely complex multiple interactions of hormones within our bodies, and is such a fundamental part of our make-up that we seldom stop to think about it. But hormones are extremely important. An awareness of the profound influence they exert on a woman's health and emotions – even her view of reality – is essential to making menopause a time of discovery rather than a source of misery. So central is the relationship of hormonal events in our bodies to how we think and feel that it would be no exaggeration to say the female endocrine system is an interface between body and spirit. Even our hopes and dreams are echoed in surges of hormones and in their shifting patterns. Changes in hormonal balance from day to day – even from moment to moment – can not only alter the way you feel emotionally, but affect your view of reality, determining whether you see life as a challenge to be met or a source of constant misery and disappointment. This is why hormonal imbalances create such emotional and spiritual agonies in women, such as those associated with PMS or menopausal symptoms. The emotional aspects of a woman's hormonal interactions are all too often forgotten in contemporary Western society. Instead of regarding our changes in mood and personality as natural, we tend to think we should always be the same, always rational, reliable, reasonable and steady. Meanwhile, synthetic hormones – drugs with potentially devastating side-effects – continue to be doled out to us from puberty onwards, with no respect for our cyclic nature and little concern for the long-term consequences these chemicals can have on our health and emotions.

How Hormones Work

The interactions between hormones in the female body are so complicated that many are still not understood by science. Bear with me while we explore the basics. Some of what follows may sound just a bit like one of those children's manuals on sex, but it really is vital to understand how the main steroid hormones in your body act and interact if you are to take control of your life, maximise your health and make menopause an adventure instead of a catalogue of misery.

Hormones perform many tasks. Some help to produce or

store energy, trigger growth, or balance blood sugar; others affect your water balance or your metabolic rate. Still others regulate respiration, cell metabolism or neural activity. Classified by their chemical structure, hormones can be either polypeptides or proteins, phenol derivatives or steroids. It is the task of the steroid hormones – from the oestrogens and progesterone to DHEA, cortisol, aldosterone and others – that we are mostly concerned with here. They regulate sex and reproduction as well as balancing brain chemistry and helping the body to handle stress without succumbing to illness.

Although they are produced in small doses, steroids pack a big punch. Each is highly specific in its actions. A hormone will excite only the particular cells it is designed to affect. How this happens is one of Nature's cleverest tricks. A molecule of a certain hormone – progesterone or DHEA, for example – has a unique shape. It will be ignored by all receptor molecules (keyholes on the cells) as it travels through the body until it is at last recognised by the particular receptor molecule with which it is meant to connect. Into this receptor site, and into it alone, the hormone molecule fits perfectly – just the way a key does in its lock. So powerful are a hormone's actions that your body needs to make only minute quantities of each as they are required. For instance, at any moment there may be as little as one molecule of a particular hormone to every fifty thousand million other molecules in your bloodstream.

The body's production of hormones and the way in which the relationship between them is continuously adjusted rely on complex interactions involving your pituitary gland (a tiny gland at the base of your brain) and your hypothalamus (often called 'the master gland'), as well as other glands such as the adrenals. In addition to producing sex-related hormones such as the oestrogens, the adrenals manufacture other important steroids including cortisol and aldosterone. Cortisol's main function is to look after blood sugar levels, on which energy depends, while aldosterone oversees potassium and magnesium excretion and sodium retention and influences both blood pressure and fluid retention.

Moon Cycles and Ovarian Rites

First, let's look at the hormonal duet which is played by the major sex hormones oestrogen and progesterone, not in your forties or fifties when you are most likely to be faced with symptoms that can cause you grief, but long before. For it is the way you live during the menstrual years – what you eat, how you use your body, what medications you take or don't take – that can set the stage for a trouble-free natural menopause.

Only since the late nineteenth century have women's menstrual cycles – the menses – been investigated scientifically. The name 'menses' also comes from a Greek word meaning 'month'. It in turn is derived from an even older word meaning 'moon'. Quite literally, the menses is the period of waxing and waning between one new moon and the next. Once menstruation begins at puberty, the ebbs and flows which a girl's body goes through each month have one major goal – child-bearing. And its success depends greatly upon the two major steroids – the oestrogens and progesterone – working in close communication with her body's major control centres: the pituitary and hypothalamus.

For the first eight to eleven days of the menstrual cycle a woman's ovaries make lots of oestrogen. Within the ovary itself are little things called follicles – partially developed eggs. One of these will be released each month in the hope of meeting up with a sperm and creating an embryo. It is oestrogen which prepares the bloody lining of the uterus and causes the follicle to develop in the ovary, bringing it to the surface of the ovary and preparing for its release. The word 'oestrogen', like the names of hormones produced in a woman's body which belong to this family – oestrone, oestradiol, and oestriol – comes from *oestrus*, a Greek word meaning 'frenzy', 'heat', or 'fertility'. It is oestrogen which brings about the changes that take place at puberty: the growth of breasts, the development of a girl's reproductive system, the reshaping of her body. It also alters her vaginal secretions, making them more viscous and less watery, and it causes her body temperature to rise at the time of ovulation, by about one degree.

Peaks and Falls

From day one until about day thirteen of a woman's menstrual cycle the level of progesterone in her body is very, very low. Yet, from the point at which a follicle is released, it rises dramatically until day twenty-one to twenty-three, at which point it begins to fall, reaching its lowest level as menstruation begins around day twenty-eight. In addition to maintaining the lining of the womb and reducing activity in the other ovary, the progesterone produced each month travels to other parts of a woman's body to fulfil other roles. For example, it protects her from the side-effects of oestrogen, helping to prevent breast cancer, water and salt retention, high blood pressure, and depression. Progesterone also brings surges of libido. You still hear a few so-called experts say that oestrogen increases libido. But think about it. Which hormone would you rely on for sex-drive – oestrogen which is present before the egg is made, or progesterone, which is produced after the egg is released and is ready for fertilisation? Libido increases with progesterone surges. When the rhythmic cycle of oestrogen and progesterone during the lunar month gets out of sync (and many factors in modern life can cause this), all sorts of things can go wrong, from infertility to PMS, depression, bloating, endometriosis and fibroids. The oestrogens and progesterone have their characteristic roles to play and for a woman to be healthy they must balance each other.

Progesterone is the mother of many other hormones. It can eventually be turned not only into various oestrogens but also into cortisol – the anti-inflammatory hormone – and into other steroids such as corticosterone or aldosterone, which have equally important jobs to do. These conversions happen as a result of slight alterations in the shape of a molecule caused by the actions of enzymes, each of which carries out a specific task. These conversions can only take place if the molecules on which the enzyme is acting 'fit' precisely into its structure. All of these changes, created by the magic of enzymes, occur in the presence of vitamins and minerals such as magnesium, zinc, and B_6.

The names and chemical transformations from one steroid to another are not important to remember. What is important is that you get some sense of just how complex hormone synthesis and interactions can be. Yet all this does not even begin to take into account the myriad pathways by which these steroid hormones interact with other hormones, master central mechanisms within the hypothalamus and pituitary, and affect our emotions, while our emotions, in turn, affect our hormones.

Sabotage

The action of synthetic hormone drugs can wreak havoc on the richly textured harmony of the hormone system. Although these drugs resemble your body's home-made hormones, the shapes of their molecules have been altered slightly by adding extra atoms here or there at unusual positions. It is this that enables them to qualify as patentable drugs, i.e. drugs which can earn their manufacturers money. However, unlike the natural hormones which they attempt to mimic, these drugs – oestrogens and 'progestogens' – are end-product molecules. Your body cannot use them to make other hormones; they are completely foreign to the human body, and unlike Nature's own steroids, they cannot be augmented or diminished as necessary to maintain hormonal balance. Also, they cannot easily be eliminated when their levels get too high.

Although the synthetics can bind with the receptor sites of the hormones they are made to mimic, they don't fit as well as our own natural hormones. Drug-based oestrogens and progestagens in contraceptives and HRT cocktails can significantly disrupt a woman's normal hormonal cycles by introducing foreign elements into her body. So, although in the short term they can provide birth control or quell heavy bleeding in a menopausal woman, in the long run they sabotage hormonal and emotional balance. Unfortunately, this is not something you will find described in the Merck index, which warns doctors of a drug's side-effects, however. The spiritual and emotional aspects of health and healing tend to be all but forgotten in most twentieth-century medical practice characterised by drug-based treatment. In the Western world we are trained to take a pill for whatever ails us. The concept that synthetic drugs should be avoided can be a little difficult for some women to accept, especially if they are well educated, if they have been urged from puberty to rely on oral contraceptives – and even told they are irresponsible if they don't – or if they have been filled with fear that if they don't take HRT as menopause approaches their lives are going to fall apart.

Friends and Lovers

Quite apart from their biochemical actions, hormones, rather like people, have highly individual 'personalities'. To bio-chemists, the personalities of the oestrogens and progesterone will always remain a mystery. They are interested only in their molecular configurations. But many women come to know these personalities well, by allowing intuition and instinct to be their teachers. When progesterone is surging through the body, a woman can feel high. Provided her body is producing enough of this steroid she is likely to feel great. The senses are acute when progesterone is running. Smells smell sweeter, or more unpleasant. Touching, sensing, tasting and hearing are all richer experiences than usual. Under the influence of progesterone, women feel the desire to do something, to create something, to work in the garden, to dance, sing a song, or make love. Sometimes progesterone surges can feel like falling in love. They can bring feelings of balanced wellbeing together with excitement, the urge to explore new worlds and to try new things. This can happen during the *luteal* phase of the menstrual cycle, after ovulation, but it becomes far more intense when she is pregnant. It is her high levels of progesterone that make a woman feel on top of the world during the last months of pregnancy. At this time the placenta churns out an amazing 300 to 400 milligrams of the steroid, while during the luteal phase of her menstrual cycle it will have only been producing 20 milligrams or so a day.

I suspect that in those women who get pregnant time and again, and who so love the whole experience, you are likely to find high progesterone levels. You also find them in women who have trouble-free menstruation. Sadly, the opposite is true too: women in whom progesterone levels are low – as they are in a growing number of women who have been subjected to manufactured hormones and, living in an increasingly polluted world, have become oestrogen-dominant – never seem to feel well, even during pregnancy. Many have all sorts of troubles with their female organs and cycles, including PMS.

When Oestrogens Flow

The oestrogens have quite a different character. When oestrogens peak in the menstrual cycle just before the 'fall' of ovulation, a woman feels less independent. She is more willing to adjust herself to the needs of others. She is more inclined to see herself in relation to men instead of as a woman in her own right. When the oestrogens are running, a woman wants to attract a mate not so much to draw him into her body as to have him comfort, admire and care for her. Her ovaries seem to be smiling – 'whatever you want, I'm happy to give,' they seem to say. A few women who are naturally high oestrogen producers feel dependent on others for approval and for the definition of their being. While such an experience can be lovely and make a woman feel highly 'feminine', it can also go too far. However, when menopause finally arrives and oestrogen levels drop dramatically, these women often find, to their surprise and delight, that for the first time in their lives they begin to feel complete in themselves – as though they don't need anybody else to validate their lives. Provided they are otherwise well, menopause can be sheer joy for such women, in the sense of freedom it brings, once they get over the shock of being such a 'different person'.

The reproductive hormonal menstrual cycle of a woman between puberty and menopause is a superbly ordered natural work of art. It becomes so much a part of our lives that unless we have some particular difficulties with PMS or fertility we hardly give it thought – that is, until things begin to alter. Once they do begin – in most women some time between the ages of forty and fifty – they usually change gradually, until finally a woman senses that something deep in her being has shifted. Such feelings herald the coming of menopause, the third phase of a woman's life.

Take Control

There is mounting dissatisfaction among women at continually being told that drug-based HRT is the only answer to mid-life depression, hot flushes, loss of sexual appetite and early ageing, probably because such advice runs counter to our deepest intuition. For many who have followed it, the use of hormonal drugs has ultimately created more problems than it solved. There is also a growing realisation among women that osteoporosis – female plague of the late twentieth century – can be stopped and that we as women need only to understand what causes this galloping consumption of our bones and take effective action to stop it. At the same time more and more women in mid-life instinctively feel it should not be necessary to fill their bodies with drugs to keep them from falling apart nor to plaster their faces with expensive cosmetics to keep their skin from looking like an alligator's hide. Although scientific information and simple do-it-yourself techniques for natural menopause are readily available, they are not much promoted, simply because most are uncommercial – there is little money to be made from them. Many women also deeply resent the negative image of the post-menopausal woman and the loss of respect for the female that Western society promulgates. Finally, women all over the world are increasingly determined not only to tap their own wisdom and dream their dreams but – as their child-bearing years come to an end – to turn their dreams into reality.

In recent years we have witnessed a revolution in pregnancy and natural childbirth. Women were once dazzled by high-tech medical intervention at birth and all too willing to surrender their bodies to epidurals, episiotomies and foetal-monitoring equipment, but in the last twenty years this has changed. We have witnessed a demand for natural childbirth, breast-feeding and good mother–child bonding. And there has developed a growing willingness among medical practitioners and government agencies to provide them. It is women themselves, led by a handful of visionary doctors and thinkers, who have helped to make the world aware of the importance of natural childbirth and who have encouraged other women to insist upon it, for their own welfare and that of their children.

Bloodless Revolution

We are poised at the brink of a new revolution. This time the revolution in women's natural health care focuses on the years just before, during and after menopause. This gentle yet persistent uprising takes its impetus from two sources: first, from an urgent demand among women themselves for profound change; second, from a group of visionaries, pioneers and trailblazers who present us with the means for bringing it about. A growing number of scientists and doctors now seriously challenge the wisdom of established medical practice – the doling out of potent drug-based hormones from puberty onwards and the widespread propaganda which accompanies it. Such practices, they say, are seriously undermining the long-term health and fertility of women as well as poisoning the environment. These visionaries, scientists and experts are not trying to damn HRT, but rather to put it in perspective. They maintain that while it may be useful for short periods in the small number of women who actually need extra oestrogen, for most women the use of drug-based hormones is costly in financial and physical terms. Meanwhile, at grass-roots level more and more women are speaking against the use of hormone drugs in the 'treatment' of menopause, drugs that have been shown to have harmful side-effects ranging from cancer to thrombosis.

The reason for such protests is simple. It is our bodies which have to bear the consequences. We sense that whatever menopause may be, it most certainly is not a disease requiring urgent treatment. The guidance we need, as women, is already available so long as we are willing to look far and wide enough for it and provided we adamantly refuse to buy into the fear-mongering, financially exploitative system that would make every menopausal woman a 'patient' for the rest of her life. Groups of women in Canada, the United States, Britain, Australia, South Africa and New Zealand are already demanding another way. They want to know about herbs and homoeopathic remedies. They are rediscovering traditional, natural alternatives supported by reliable scientific findings and current clinical use. They are also exploring how natural hormones and 'smart drugs' can be used to balance brain and mood, to heighten immunity and to slow down ageing. They are demanding methods of self-care that take into account how mind and body interact, and reject symptomatic treatments which carry the threat of dangerous side-effects. The time has come, they insist, for us to stop thinking of ourselves as victims – victims of cancer, of PMS, menopausal trauma or anything else. When you see yourself in the role of a victim, nothing can help you. The first step to a natural menopause is to change your perception of it. Stop thinking of yourself as a victim of symptoms you can do nothing about, learn how to help yourself, and you will reclaim your power. Menopause is the time to assert your right to freedom.

Step Two
Get Savvy

WE LIVE in a world where it is easy for a woman's bio-chemistry to become distorted by declining physical activity, the proliferation of highly processed convenience foods, the devastating effects of environmental pollution, and the rise of a whole new – as yet largely unrecognised – phenomenon known as *oestrogen-dominance*. An awareness of the profound influence they exert on a woman's health and emotions is essential. The second step towards a natural menopause is to get savvy. To defeat the enemy, you need to know what it is.

Perils of Pathology

For too many women in the Western world, their first experience of menopause is a physical complaint for which they seek medical advice: endometriosis, fibroid tumours, depression, or the kind of persistent excessive bleeding that can make a woman weak with anaemia and weary of struggle. If surgery is not seen to be the answer, often a woman is led to believe that HRT is. Even today, just about everyone will leap to the conclusion that a menopausal woman needs oestrogen. Many women (and their doctors) still believe that when menstruation finally ceases a woman's oestrogen production falls to nothing. They also think that it is oestrogen which keeps skin young-looking and sexuality flourishing.

A woman's oestrogen production does not cease at menopause. Only oestrogen production in her ovaries stops, preventing the monthly build-up of the womb lining in preparation for pregnancy. This is also why menstruation no longer takes place. Provided her body is in good balance and she is healthy, the oestrogen she now makes in her fat cells, in her liver, and in her adrenals is all she will ever need. What does cease, however – or pretty nearly ceases – as soon as menopause arrives (if not earlier) is the production of progesterone. It can fall to near zero. Because progesterone is a precursor of so many other steroid hormones, when the body's production of it ceases, or when oestrogen-dominance gets out of hand, other hormones – from sex hormones to corticosteroids – are not produced adequately either. Some of the hormones of which progesterone is a precursor are brain chemicals which influence the way we think and feel. Others are needed by the body to protect against inflammation and early ageing or to sustain libido. The absence of sufficient quantities of these can produce aches and pains in the joints, and chronic fatigue as well as depression, hot flushes and anxiety. It can also be a prime cause of the emotional upsets which many women experience in mid-life. Such experiences are most assuredly not a natural part of growing older. They are signs that a woman's hormonal balance needs to be improved.

Chemical Seas

Most of the health problems associated with menopause are the result of the way a woman's major reproductive hormones have become unbalanced by twentieth-century pollution. The *leitmotif* running through almost all of the 'menopausal horrors' – mood swings, night sweats, fibroids, PMS, endometriosis, breast cancer – is *oestrogen-dominance*. Oestrogen-dominance means high levels of oestrogen or oestrogen-like chemicals in a woman's body, coupled with a relative lack of progesterone. Oestrogen-dominance has developed for many reasons, including the widespread use of oestrogen-based oral contraceptives and the exponential spread in our environment of chemicals which are oestrogen mimics. We are, say environmental scientists, immersed in a rising sea of petrochemical derivatives. They are in our air, our foods and our water. These chemicals include pesticides and herbicides as well as various plastics which are capable of mimicking the action of oestrogen in the body. Thousands of miles from where they were used to spray crops, they can be found in quantity in the fat of Arctic seals. Gradually, over the years, we accumulate these toxins in the fat of our own bodies.

Hidden Danger

Of the thousands of oestrogens and oestrogen-like chemicals which appear to be responsible for the mounting incidence of oestrogen-dominance in our culture, none are as sinister as the *xenoestrogens*. The word *xeno* means 'strange' or 'foreign'. Xenoestrogen is the name given to the widespread environmental pollutants and chemicals that mimic the effects of a woman's own natural oestrogens and undermine the balance of oestrogens and progesterone in her body. Because xenoestrogens are taken up by oestrogen receptor sites in the body, and because the hormones in the body interact with its organs and systems as well as with each other in highly complex and interdependent ways, they can disrupt the workings of the body as a whole.

This group of environmental toxins includes hundreds of chemicals: the *polycarbonated plastics* found in our baby bottles and water jugs; the *polychlorinated biphenyls* (PCBs) used in the manufacture of electronics; highly poisonous pesticides such as DDT and its even more toxic cousin DDE to *dieldrin, toxaphene, mirex, heptachlor* and *kepone* as well as a multitude of other herbicides and pesticides, all of which have an ability to mimic natural oestrogen. Even the breakdown products from many common detergents, and chlorine compounds now used to bleach paper, can do this. Our world is full of plastics – containers we use every day to store leftovers in the refrigerator or cook food in the microwave, disposable cups we drink coffee from, bottles our mineral water comes in. Few companies that manufacture plastics know whether or not their products slough off oestrogen-like molecules.

Locks and Keys

Although the use of a number of PCBs has been restricted in many industrialised countries, like DDT and a few pesticides known to be highly toxic, the products of their breakdown persist in the environment for decades. Hormones used in birth control and in hormone replacement are other forms of oestrogens foreign to the human system. As endocrinologist David Feldman from Stanford University says: 'It is very possible – and it is frightening – that we may be drowning in a sea of oestrogens.' Most forms of oestrogens, natural or chemical, are capable of bringing about biochemical changes in the body, because they are able to attach themselves to receptor sites within the body's cells. Unfortunately, oestrogen receptor sites are not particularly choosy. Fraudulent oestrogens in pesticides and other chemicals can hook on to them just as easily as the real thing.

Cell receptor sites act like a lock which needs a hormone or vitamin 'key' to open them. For a long time scientists believed that each lock would open only when presented with the exact molecular key intended for it. Recently, however, they have discovered that many foreign chemicals are also capable of opening up oestrogen receptors. Some oestrogen-mimic molecules fit into the receptor keyholes but won't fully unlock them, so they don't trigger normal activity on a cellular level. Others behave like poorly cut keys: sometimes they turn the lock, sometimes they don't. A third group act like skeleton keys: they appear to fit perfectly into a receptor and fully unlock its gene action, yet bring devastating effects in their wake. Once locked on to a receptor site, oestrogen mimics can fool the body into turning off certain biochemical pathways. This can have consequences including the development of cancers of the breast and womb, endometriosis, infertility, and changes in the reproductive and hormone systems not only of adults but also of unborn children.

Secrets of Oestrogen

In order to grasp how xenoestrogens affect the body it is important to remember how the natural oestrogens work. Although people commonly refer to '*oestrogen*' in the singular, this hormone is not a single compound. It is a group of many different compounds, each with different characteristics and actions. 'Oestrogen' is the collective name used to describe all natural and artificial chemicals which are able to trigger *oestrus*, the release of an egg in a woman. Oestrogen is secreted primarily by the ovarian follicles of menstruating women. During pregnancy it is also secreted by the placenta. To be absolutely accurate, there is no such thing as 'oestrogen'; however the word is used to describe many compounds – both those that occur naturally, in our foods and in our bodies, and those that are synthetically manufactured, either as hormone drugs or petrochemical derivatives – which exert an oestrogenic effect on the body.

There are three major kinds of oestrogens made in the human body: *oestradiol* – the most common and the most potent, *oestriol*, and *oestrone*. Men too produce oestrogen but in much smaller quantities than we do. When puberty arrives oestrogens in a girl encourage the development of breasts and the expansion of the uterus. After that they help to regulate the menstrual cycle and play other important roles, such as helping to maintain bone mass and keeping blood cholesterol levels in check. When excessive quantities of oestrogen (regardless of source) are present in a young woman's body, they will burn out her ovaries and undermine fertility. It is this phenomenon which many eco-scientists believe to be largely responsible for the rapidly decreasing fertility of Western women. Many women have been taught that after menopause a woman's body stops making oestrogen. This common error ultimately leads to an even greater untruth: that menopause is an 'oestrogen deficiency disease'. After menopause oestrogen continues to be made in a woman's body, but in much smaller quantities.

Growing Problem

Each year brings further evidence that women in industrialised countries are suffering from overexposure to oestrogen mimics. In 1960 the chances of a woman developing breast cancer were only one in twenty. Today one in nine women are statistically destined to get the disease. Only about thirty per cent of women who get breast cancer now are in what are considered high-risk groups: women who reach puberty early, who don't breast-feed or breast-feed for only a limited period, who come from a family with a history of breast cancer, or who have their first pregnancy late in life. To make things even more complicated, not all oestrogens or oestrogen-like substances exert the negative effect on the body that oestrogen drugs and xenoestrogens can. In the same way that medicine now recognises that there is a good-guy cholesterol and a bad-guy cholesterol in relation to protecting the body from heart disease, so there are 'good' and 'bad' oestrogens. Recent research has shown that a number of weaker natural oestrogen-like ingredients in foods actually help to protect us against cancer of the breast and reproductive system. When these beneficial *phyto-oestrogens* bind to oestrogen receptor sites, they can not only supply an alternative form of natural oestrogen where needed but, by taking up her oestrogen receptor sites, they may protect the woman from the xenoestrogens in her environment which are continually trying to key into them.

The old saying 'these days a man is only half his grandfather' may actually be true. Danish endocrinologist Niels Skakkebaek, a researcher at the Rigshospital in Copenhagen, reported in 1992 that there has been a fifty per cent drop in sperm counts world-wide. During this same period the incidence of testicular cancer has tripled in many countries, while that of prostate cancer has doubled. In Germany, researchers have recently discovered that women with endometriosis – the condition which very commonly occurs in women over forty where the lining of the womb painfully proliferates – have significantly higher levels of PCBs in their bodies than women without the disease. Seventy years ago only twenty-one cases of endometriosis had been reported in the world. Now, there are more than five million cases in the United States alone.

DDE-Sexed Alligators

Not long ago in Lake Apopka in Florida, wildlife biologists discovered that vast numbers of alligator eggs were failing to hatch. In those that did, the male alligators had abnormally small penises – seventy-five per cent shorter than average. Almost certainly, say scientists investigating the phenomenon, this is the result of residual concentrations of DDE from a lake-side spill many years before. Following up this hypothesis, Louis J. Guillette, wildlife endocrinologist at the University of Florida, experimented with DDE xenoestrogens. He discovered that painting alligator eggs with the same doses of DDE which are present in the lake – such low doses that they can only be measured in parts per billion – brings about the same reproductive problems in laboratory animals. Only ten per cent of the treated eggs hatch and most of these animals turn out to be female.

Plague of Plagues

What appears to be happening is that a strange and potentially highly dangerous marriage is taking place between the increase of oestrogen-mimicking chemicals in the environment and the rise in various oestrogens prescribed medically to women. It is probably out of this union that oestrogen-dominance has developed. The oestrogens and progesterone in a woman's body must balance each other for a woman to remain healthy. In many of us they are becoming more and more out of kilter. As a result we are now seeing a widespread rise in many diseases and symptoms for which – with a strange irony – doctors are prescribing more oestrogen. Here are a few of the ways in which oestrogen-dominance can manifest:

- When oestrogen is not balanced by progesterone it can produce weight gain, headache, bad temper, chronic fatigue and loss of interest in sex – all of which are part of the clinically recognised pre-menstrual syndrome or PMS.

- Not only has it been well established that oestrogen-dominance encourages the development of breast cancer, the action of oestrogen also stimulates breast tissue and can in time trigger fibrocystic breast disease, a condition which wanes when natural progesterone is added to a woman's body to balance the oestrogen.

- By definition, excess oestrogen implies a progesterone deficiency. This in turn leads to a decrease in the rate of new bone formation in a woman's body – the prime cause of osteoporosis.

- Oestrogen-dominance increases the risk of fibroids. One of the interesting facts about fibroids – often remarked on by doctors – is that, regardless of their size, fibroids commonly shrink once menopause arrives and a woman's ovaries are no longer making oestrogen.

- In oestrogen-dominant menstruating women in whom progesterone is not peaking and falling in a normal way each month, the ordered shedding of the womb lining doesn't take place. Menstruation cycles become irregular.

- Endometrial cancer – cancer of the womb – develops only where there is oestrogen-dominance. Some of the artificial progestagens may also help to prevent it, which is why a growing number of doctors no longer give oestrogen without combining it with a progestogen drug during HRT.

- Water retention and an increase in sodium levels in the body which predispose a woman to high blood pressure or hypertension, frequently occur with oestrogen-dominance. This can also be a side-effect of taking a progestogen.

- The risk of stroke and heart disease increases dramatically when a woman is oestrogen-dominant.

Go to the Source

So potentially dangerous is oestrogen-dominance that it is essential we communicate information about it both to other women of all ages and to our doctors. It is also important that we put pressure on our politicians and government leaders to tighten controls over the chemicals that are allowed to be used in the environment. Scientists throughout the Western world are working to identify the specific agents responsible for the increase in xenoestrogens in our environment. However, we are constantly exposed to so many chemicals which exhibit an oestrogenic characteristic that this task may turn out to be as difficult as finding the proverbial needle in the haystack. Some researchers suspect that *ethynylestradiol* (EE) – the primary oestrogenic compound in birth control pills – plays a major role. Because EE in the urine of women on the pill is able to pass through water treatment plants, it ends up in our drinking water. To test the effect of EE and other oestrogens on wildlife, researchers raised fish in aquariums which had dilute concentrations either of EE or oestradiol, the primary oestrogen in the the animal kingdom. They found that even concentrations of EE as low as 0.1 nanograms per litre of water have a significant effect. Researchers concluded that EE is one of the most potent of biological active molecules. At the Fish and Wildlife Services in Atlanta, Georgia, scientists have since issued a prohibition on the use of oestrogenic chemicals, including pesticides, in the more than a hundred wildlife refuges in the south-western United States managed by the federal government.

Little information about the mounting effects of xenoestrogens and oestrogen-dominance in women has even begun to filter down to the general public. Neither has it yet been made easily available to the busy doctors to whom women suffering from PMS or menopause-related symptoms turn for help. That's the bad news. The good news is that information about xenoestrogens is beginning to be available in most countries, as are natural, non-drug over-the-counter products such as progesterone creams, and also herbs and plant products that are safe and effective.

Forgotten Hormone

An understanding of what progesterone is and how it works is central to the revolution in natural menopause. Among this hormone's many attributes – which include restoring emotional balance, enhancing a woman's ability to handle stress, and improving the look of her skin – is an ability to do what most medical science still considers impossible: reverse osteoporosis. Exciting as all this may sound, progesterone is not some miracle substance; nor is it a new-fangled alternative to HRT. It is simply a forgotten piece of the menopause puzzle.

Antagonist to the collective oestrogen, progesterone is the single steroid female hormone – one specific molecule – made by the *corpus luteum*. The corpus luteum is the yellow granular mass in the ovary formed each month after an egg has been released. Whereas oestrogen is the major female reproductive hormone during the first half of a woman's menstrual cycle, progesterone is the most important hormone during the second half. Progesterone promotes changes in the womb lining that make the uterus ready for implantation by a fertilised egg. When a woman is pregnant, the placenta takes over her body's production of progesterone, which now increases ten- or twenty-fold – sometimes more – above its previous level. During pregnancy progesterone helps the womb to hold the baby safely until it is ready to be born. When women miscarry, it is often because their bodies do not produce enough progesterone, especially during the early stages of pregnancy. Progesterone, and plants containing chemicals from which the body can make this hormone, have been used throughout history to arrest threatened miscarriages. In addition, it is also the high level of progesterone synthesised during pregnancy that makes many women feel and look so well – often better than at any other time in their lives – during the last few months before giving birth.

Progesterone or not Progesterone?

Surrounding the word 'progesterone' are many misconceptions, and they take a bit of sorting out. For a start, the word 'progesterone' tends to be used erroneously and collectively – by doctors, researchers and the media alike – to describe not the natural hormone itself, but one or more of the *progestogens*. These are synthetic progesterone-analogues, such as the widely used drugs *Provera*, *Duphaston* and *Primalut*. Together with one or more forms of oestrogen, progestogens – also called *progestins* or *gestins* – are incorporated into contraceptive pills and HRT. You will often hear doctors say that 'progesterone does this or that'. But when you actually pin them down and get them to clarify what they are talking about, ninety-nine times out of a hundred you will find that they are using the word wrongly, to describe not the natural hormone progesterone, but rather one of these synthetic analogues.

The effects of natural and synthetic hormones on the body differ enormously. The synthetics do not match the body's chemistry, so the body is not equipped to metabolise them properly. Taking a progestogen can inhibit ovulation in a menstruating woman. It can also suppress her body's production of its own natural progesterone and trigger other negative side-effects. You will find them listed at length in the manual your doctor refers to when prescribing drugs. Progesterone itself, on the other hand, has none of these. The use of synthetic progestogen in HRT can all too often aggravate some of the problems a doctor is trying to treat, making women moody, irritable and bad-tempered. Natural progesterone, by contrast, tends to make women feel calm and stable. In Europe and North America a growing number of doctors and women who have used natural progesterone obtained from plant sources report that it also banishes hot flushes, re-establishes fertility, eliminates PMS and reverses osteoporosis. But, since the natural hormone and the various progestogens so often get lumped together in common medical parlance, progesterone is frequently blamed for negative effects which it doesn't cause.

The Colour of Money

Why would pharmaceutical manufacturers forgo a perfectly natural hormone, like progesterone which is chemically identical to the body's own hormone and offers all these benefits without any risk to safety or negative side-effects, choosing instead to market products which are synthetic and which, because they are foreign to the body, carry serious potential side-effects? The reason is a simple one. It lies behind the continuing insistence of the medical-industrial complex that drug-based HRT is the treatment of choice for just about every peri-menopausal, menopausal and post-menopausal complaint you can imagine. Once you have synthesised a compound in the laboratory – once you have made a unique molecule, one which is not found in nature – you have a drug that you can patent and own. As soon as a company patents such a compound it can control its sales and its price so that it cannot be undersold. In fact, nobody else can sell the drug at all. This is what the pharmaceutical business is all about. And a very big business it is, with enormous profits.

Selling drugs is a very different kettle of fish from selling herbs, nutritional supplements or a generic hormone like progesterone. Pharmaceutical companies can sell genuine therapeutic substances such as vitamin C, vitamin D or natural progesterone, but will never be able to acquire a patent on them since these are all compounds obtainable from nature and anybody else can sell them too. To do further medical research on a new use for a compound like progesterone would cost hundreds of thousands of pounds – as much as the research into a new drug. If any manufacturer were to undertake such research and spend the huge sums of money necessary to establish that progesterone is beneficial, the money they invested would be largely wasted, because their competitors could then produce the same product and reap all the financial rewards without ever having spent a penny. So pharmaceutical companies who manufacture contraceptives and HRT drugs choose instead to grow massive quantities of the Mexican wild yam, extract its diosgenin, turn it into progesterone and then, by altering the molecule further, produce a unique and patentable synthetic drug. Meanwhile, natural progesterone never has been – and it seems unlikely that it ever will be – produced by a large drug company. For it will never be a patentable commodity from which a pharmaceutical manufacturer can derive big profits.

The Champions

For the past twenty years, while the high-powered medical world extolled the virtues of oestrogen drugs and HRT, John Lee, a country doctor in northern California, diligently researched the actions of natural progesterone. When he began to apply his knowledge of this remarkable hormone – available in many countries without prescription in the form of a cream – Lee discovered that women who use it are able to eliminate a myriad of menstrual and pre-menstrual problems and menopausal complaints for which conventional medical science still has no answers. In some cases natural progesterone has even been shown to help to make barren women fertile. It was Lee who a few years ago coined the term 'oestrogen-dominance'. Oestrogen-dominance is relatively easy to correct once you know how. And correcting it when it has occurred in the body brings enormous benefits to a woman's overall health and life.

Lee's Story

In 1976 – the heyday of oestrogen replacement in the United States – a general consensus conference was held at the Mayo Clinic. The doctors gathered there from around the world decided that oestrogen – the only hormone then used to treat osteoporosis and menopause-related symptoms – should no longer be given on its own, since more and more of the women on oestrogen replacement were developing cancer of the uterus. By the time of the Mayo conference it had been well established that giving excess oestrogen as oestrogen replacement to women with a history of breast cancer is highly dangerous because in some women the proliferative character of oestrogen reactivates cancerous growth. John Lee did not know what to prescribe for his women patients who had osteoporosis but were already at risk of developing cancer.

In 1979 Lee heard a talk given by one of the trailblazers in the natural menopause revolution, Dr Ray Peat. In the lecture Peat pointed out that the medical profession had virtually forgotten that natural progesterone exists. He said that progesterone is easy to obtain, and that it can be derived from many plants. Unlike the progestogens, progesterone has no negative side-effects, said Peat. It is even included in the formulas of certain cosmetics because it is so good for skin. Peat felt strongly that doctors should consider using progesterone in their treatment of women patients. Peat's words rang bells for John Lee. He contacted the biochemist and asked for all his research references. Later, ploughing through scientific papers, Lee discovered that Peat was right. There had indeed been masses of research into the uses of natural progesterone right from the early 1900s up to around 1960. After that, with the development of the synthetic progestogens, little further research was carried out into the natural hormone.

John Lee spent a long time gathering Ray Peat's references. He discovered many new ones, too. Everything Peat had said about progesterone seemed to be true. No one had ever found it to cause a negative side-effect. As far as its benefits were concerned, they turned out to be far greater than Lee had imagined. Progesterone helps the thyroid hormone to do its job properly, for instance. It protects against the waterlogging which excess oestrogen can cause and against the retention of sodium which results in waterlogging. It also helps to keep cell membranes intact, so that they are not easily damaged by viruses or toxic substances from the air we breathe, the water we drink, and the food we eat. Progesterone even has an anti-ageing effect on skin. It is a natural antidepressant and can restore lost libido. All of this sounded pretty good to Lee, so he suggested to his women patients who suffered from osteoporosis – whether or not they were taking oestrogen replacement – that they go to their pharmacy or their health food store, buy a jar of progesterone cream and try it for themselves.

Leap in the Dark

About that same time a new technique for measuring bone mineral density had been developed: *photon absorptiometry*. Photons – which are seen as a kind of orange or pinkish glow – are transmitted through skin and flesh, bouncing off when they hit bone. The number of molecules that bounce off is then calibrated to indicate the extent of mineral deposits which the beams are hitting. The new technique enabled technicians to measure the bone mineral density of any woman to within ninety-six to ninety-eight per cent of absolute accuracy. It was a real breakthrough. Methods in use before the 1980s were highly inaccurate. X-rays, for instance, besides subjecting women to doses of radiation, are not able to show the degree of bone loss until it exceeds thirty per cent. And if a woman has a thirty per cent bone loss she is already terribly at risk of fracture.

Lee not only wanted to see what effect topically applied progesterone would have on women, he wanted accurate objective measurements of how progesterone, used regularly, would affect osteoporosis. So he persuaded his women patients to have bone mineral density tests done in this new way. He took measurements of their bone mineral density before they began using progesterone cream and then again at intervals afterwards, and he kept extensive records of changes observed. All his patients had to do – in addition to taking a few vitamin and minerals, watching their diet and getting a bit of exercise – was to rub a little of the progesterone cream on to their skin once or twice a day. To Lee's amazement six months to a year later not only had progesterone been able to protect these women from further bone mineral loss, it had actually improved the state of their bones and cured problems ranging from PMS to menopausal symptoms.

Simple Balance

Lee observed that the progesterone cream could eliminate the excess facial hair which some women develop as they get older, and prevent the weakening of nails and loss of hair from the head which others experience post-menopausally. Many of his women patients reported that after using the cream the hair on their heads grew thicker. Women who had relied on diuretics to prevent water retention usually didn't need them any more: progesterone is a natural diuretic. Lee frequently found that women with high blood pressure no longer needed to take their hypertension medication. Many women on thyroid medication no longer needed treatment either, since progesterone makes the thyroid gland function much more efficiently.

Lee discovered that when a woman first uses a progesterone cream it can make her temporarily more sensitive to the oestrogens in her body. This is because oestrogen and progesterone are not only antagonistic but synergistic in their actions. Alter the level of one and you affect the actions of the other. This means that some women experience temporary breast swelling, tenderness or other signs of excess oestrogens when they begin to use progesterone. However, these symptoms soon pass as their oestrogen-dominance disappears and their system rebalances itself. Lee also discovered from working with his patients that the presence of adequate progesterone in a woman's body automatically reduces her need for oestrogen. So if a doctor decides to give progesterone to a woman on oestrogen replacement he will need to cut her dose of oestrogen by at least half. She will then get all the benefits of oestrogen replacement – but in a much lower (and much safer) dose. Most women put on progesterone, however, find they need no extra oestrogen at all, since progesterone can be converted into oestrogen by the body.

Spread the News

The rest is history. Lee's discoveries about the reversal of osteoporosis using progesterone, unparalleled in medical history, are transforming women's natural health care. It had already been established that oestrogen supplementation could slow bone loss to some degree by preventing some of the breakdown of old bone. But oestrogen can do nothing to create new bone once mineral loss has taken place. Progesterone can. John Lee's work took place more than ten years ago. Since then information about his clinical studies using progesterone has been published in *The Lancet, International Clinical Nutritional Review* and *Medical Hypothesis* as well as in many other journals, magazines and even in a few books. Nevertheless, John Lee's findings remain virtually unknown in the mainstream medical community, and as yet far too few women know enough about progesterone to use it to improve their lives.

We will probably be well into the twenty-first century before the devastating effects of post-industrial environmental pollution can even begin to be measured. Our wildlife sent the first signals that something was seriously wrong. However, economic pressure from manufacturers of chemical products may prevent governments from introducing laws adequate to control the addition of new poisons to the rising sea of oestrogens around us which appears to be making us more oestrogen-dominant with each passing decade. But there is a great deal that a woman who feels respect for the wisdom of Nature and for her own body can now do to protect herself as well as the world around her. Understanding the problems is the second step to a natural menopause. The third is to start to take control of your own hormone health.

Step Three
Regenerate Your Body

A TIME of death and rebirth, menopause offers a woman an unequalled opportunity to regenerate and rejuvenate her body and in the process to transform her life, both physically and emotionally. Menopause is also a time to take stock of what works in your body and what does not, a time to begin listening to the rhythm of your body and your soul, even if – like many of us – you seem to have forgotten how, or are wondering if there is a soul to be heard. There are many tools and techniques that can help you do this – from from foods that build energy to exercise that builds strength, from herbs that balance hormones to techniques for finding out what you want in life. Now is the time to explore what they can offer.

Spring Clean

In order to make the most of these techniques, your body needs to be as clear and pollution-free as possible, otherwise much of the potential they offer for energy, emotional balance and mental clarity can be wasted. Step three to a natural menopause is a simple programme of detoxification to eliminate any toxins that may have built up over the months and years, while at the same time helping to supply the body with a good quantity of minerals, vitamins and micro-nutrients to support bodily functioning and hormonal balance.

Such a programme can be as useful to a menstruating woman who wants to maximise her energy and good looks and minimise PMS, emotional swings and other unpleasant symptoms as it can to a menopausal or post-menopausal woman who wants to regenerate her body. Deep-cleansing the body can be done in a number of ways: by spending time at a clinic where the principles of nature-cure are put into practice with deep-cleansing regimes; by carrying out a spring clean such as the one in my *Ten Day Clean-Up Plan*; or – and this is my favourite in mid-life – by making periodic use of a Miso Detox and Rebuild programme. This is most effective if carried out for at least a week at a time, but can be continued for several weeks to great advantage. During the first week of the programme it is best to stop taking any supplements you may be using except for a high-quality vitamin C supplement, which can actually help in the detoxification process. Most important of all, you need to increase your intake of pure water to one or two litres a day.

Let Food Be Your Medicine

Miso – pronounced *mee-so* – is also known as fermented soya-bean paste. It is a savoury paste made from soya beans and grain which has been cultured with *Aspergillus oryzae*, a micro-organism highly beneficial to the human body thanks to its ability to help set up virtually ideal conditions in the colon. This in turn helps with the body's manufacture of B vitamins important for energy and for protecting the body from excess stress, and for enabling a continuous elimination of the toxic waste build-up typical of a Western diet.

For generations Japanese folklore has taught that miso broth is beneficial for health and longevity. As a result, it still forms the basis of breakfast for over seventy per cent of the population of Japan. Recently, however, a number of scientific studies have been carried out to quantify the effects of taking miso regularly. Scientists have been able to identify some of the specific ways in which it benefits health. The daily use of miso has been shown to lower cholesterol, to alkalinise blood made acid by too much sugar, refined foods and meat, and to neutralise many of the negative effects of environmental pollution on our bodies. Most fascinating of all is miso's apparent ability to neutralise many of the effects of radiation, helping to prevent the free radical damage which underlies early ageing and the development of degenerative diseases from cancer to coronary heart disease.

Protect and Survive

The first indication of miso's effectiveness against radiation came from the work of Dr Shinchiro Akizuki. As director of the Saint Francis Hospital in Nagasaki, Akizuki spent his life treating 'ground zero' patients (people living close to where the atomic bomb had been dropped) and investigating the use of foods as preventative medicine. Although his team spent years near the site of the atomic explosion, neither Dr Akizuki nor his colleagues experienced the effects of radiation poisoning which devastated the lives of the people they were treating. He wondered if this may have been because he and his staff drank miso soup every day. Then, in 1972, his hypothesis was confirmed: scientists discovered that miso is rich in an alkaloid called *dipicolonic acid*, which is able to link up with molecules of heavy metals in the body such as lead, mercury, aluminium and radioactive strontium and carry them out of the body. A few years later at Japan's Cancer Research Centre, other researchers discovered that people who regularly consume miso soup have significantly lower levels of many forms of cancer and heart disease. And recently scientists at Tohoku University in Hokkaido have been able to isolate compounds in miso which appear to wipe out the carcinogenic or cancer-causing effects of many chemicals on the body. Scientists at Hiroshima University's Atomic Radioactivity Medical Lab under the direction of Professor Akihiro Ito have confirmed with animal experiments the free radical protection against radiation which the regular consumption of miso can bring. The liver cancer rate of animals not fed miso and then exposed to radiation is 100 to 200 per cent higher than those of animals that are.

Miso comes in many flavours and ranges in colour from the sweet pale tan varieties to the dark rich brown and red misos. Some misos are made from barley, others from rice or chickpeas. In texture they resemble a soft nut butter and can be spread on bread, added to soups, grain dishes and casseroles and used in salad dressings. The cornerstone of the miso diet for detoxification is the use of miso broth. The kind of miso which is best for this is organic *genmai* miso made from soya and brown rice. It is dark, rich in flavour and has a thick texture. Although the preparation of miso soup in Japan is an art in itself and makes use of their famous dashi broth and superbly cut vegetables, it is simple to put together an instant miso broth by placing a heaped teaspoon to a table-spoon of the miso in the bottom of a large cup or bowl and pouring boiling water over it. Then you can add sea vegetables such as flaked nori, spirulina flakes or other green power-houses like green barley or wheatgrass. I like to add a splash of good soya milk and sometimes a crushed clove of garlic or two. Once you break through old habit patterns that force you to look upon breakfast as a time for packaged cereals and coffee, you find that such a breakfast is not only satisfying, it also helps to keep your energy levels steady all through the morning and beyond. After a couple of weeks of drinking miso broth once or twice a day, the body's elimination processes move into top gear, enabling it gently yet inexorably to cast off all kinds of stored wastes that have been suppressing energy and interfering with the metabolic processes on which good hormonal balance depends.

The Principles

The basic principles of the Miso Detox and Rebuild are simple: first you remove all foods that can interfere with the body's natural abilities to cleanse itself. These include heavy proteins like meat, dairy products, wheat, sugar, junk fats and other highly processed items. Second, you cut out stimulants such as coffee and tea and depressants such as alcohol, which

Choose From	*Avoid*
Sprouted seeds and grains	Coffee
Organic miso	Tea
Fresh fruits	Alcohol
Fresh vegetables	Sugar or anything containing sugar
Seaweeds	Artificial colourings and flavourings
Green foods (spirulina, chlorella, green barley, wheat grass)	Convenience foods
Buckwheat and buckwheat noodles	Wheat and wheat products
Organic brown rice	Meat
Fresh seeds	Fish
Fresh nuts	Game
Soya milk	Cigarettes
Fresh herbs	Drugs
Low-salt vegetable bouillon powder	Chocolate
Soya seasonings (e.g. organic tamari)	Colas
Raw honey	Milk and milk products
Tofu	
Tempeh or soya cheese	
Legumes	
Extra virgin olive oil	
Herb teas	
Spring water	

tend to distort body energies and build up toxicity. Then you take in foods with deep-cleansing abilities, such as raw fruits and vege- tables and miso, to encourage the elimination of stored wastes from your body. Finally, you supply a high level of easily available nutrients from power foods such as sea plants, sprouted seeds and grains, and the green foods as well as low-fat, easily absorbed protein foods rich in natural hormones, such as the soya products tofu, tempeh, soya milk and miso itself (more about these in Step Four). This creates a way of eating which can be followed for a few days or several weeks, a programme designed to regenerate and rejuvenate the body at the deepest levels. While carrying out a Miso Detox and Rebuild, see the table on page 44 for foods to consume and those to avoid.

Bountiful Breakfast

Breakfast is simple and the same every day: a bowl of miso broth made by pouring boiling water over a tablespoon of organic genmai miso made from fermented brown rice and soya beans. Add one or more of the following to taste: nori flakes, mixed sea salad, flakes of organic spirulina, green barley powder, wheat grass powder, chlorella powder and (if, like me, you are a garlic fan) a crushed clove of fresh raw garlic. To this you can add a splash of soya milk if you wish.

It is important to experiment with miso broth. You will probably find that some of the green foods I have suggested adding to it will appeal to you, while others will not. You will also discover by trial and error the amounts of these foods your body needs and wants. This is likely to vary from time to time as well. You may find at the beginning that you want only the miso broth with a little soya milk by itself. That's fine. But do try to add the green foods bit by bit as you get used to this new kind of breakfast.

The other two meals of the day are interchangeable and can be adjusted to fit what is available on the menu of a restaurant when you need to eat out.

Sample Week's Menu for Miso Detox and Rebuild

	Main Meal	*Light Meal*
Monday	Grilled tofu spread with tamari. A fresh salad of raw beetroot and apple dressed with fresh orange juice and curry powder. A fresh peach.	Vegetable soup made with root vegetables, green vegetables, garlic, onions and low-salt vegetable bouillon. Melon.
Tuesday	Risotto of organic brown rice, vegetables. A salad of fresh spouted seeds or grains topped with mixed three seeds: pumpkin, sesame and sunflower. Half a grapefuit or tangerines.	Crudités with a dip made by blending organic tofu with garlic, lemon juice, seasoning and Worcester sauce. Miso broth with soba (100 per cent buck-wheat noodles – see page 76).
Wednesday	Sweet potatoes or baked yams topped with grated fresh ginger and extra virgin olive oil. Salad of grated celeriac, carrots, red pepper and black olives with olive oil and lemon dressing. Baked apple with raisins and cinnamon.	Fresh spinach, mushroom and garlic salad with dressing made by blending tofu with brown rice vinegar, garlic, vegetable bouillon powder and herbs. Fresh fruit salad.
Thursday	Baked carrots and parsnips with almonds or cashews, spread with miso. A cooked buckwheat and raw vegetable salad, including whatever fresh vegetables and sprouts are available. Slices of orange topped with raisins which have been plumped by soaking in spring water overnight.	Dairy-free muesli (see page 80). Bowl of miso broth if you like.

	Main Meal	*Light Meal*
Friday	Leek, parsnip and yellow split-pea soup to which you have added garlic, seaweeds and vegetable bouillon. Fresh cucumber slices topped with a dressing of olive oil, finely chopped onions, grated fresh ginger, slivered mushrooms and miso.	Sliced tomato and sesame seed salad with fresh basil (if available), cubes of organic tofu and crushed cloves of garlic. Dress with cider vinegar, olive oil, miso and honey.
Saturday	Tofu slices spread with miso then grilled and served with wok-fried fresh vegetables. A bunch of grapes.	Brown rice salad with chopped carrots, green onions, olives, tomatoes, parsley, celery and garlic, dressed with olive oil, lemon, sesame seeds and sprinkled with toasted, crumbled seaweed.
Sunday	Scrambled tofu with green salad made from Chinese leaves, herbs, celery, green pepper, spring onions and rocket. Half a melon filled with blueberries or strawberries.	Barley pilaff salad with miso sauce.* Cook and cool the barley and mix with finely chopped raw vegetables. Almond milk made in a blender from 1/2 cup of blanched almonds, raw honey, spring water, and pure vanilla essence.

* For miso sauce: 1 1/2 cups water, 2 tbsp arrowroot, 1/2 cup miso, juice of 1 lemon, 6 tbsp apple concentrate. Mix half the water with the fruit concentrate and the miso in a food processor until thoroughly blended. Mix arrowroot into a small amount of the remaining water and blend, adding more and more water until all the water is used. Heat on a medium heat, stirring briskly, until all the starch gels. Remove from the heat and stir in the miso mixture. Mix thoroughly.

Secrets of Water

When it comes to regenerating and rejuvenating the body, water is the most important nutrient of all. It is the stuff from which your blood, your cells, your muscles, and even your bones are mostly made. A healthy person who weighs 65 kilos (143 lb) carries about 40 litres (8–9 gallons) of water around: 25 litres (5^1/2 gallons) inside the cells, 15 litres (3 gallons) outside, including 5 litres (1 gallon) in the blood. Let yourself become dehydrated, and the chemical reactions in your cells become sluggish. Also, your body cannot build new tissue efficiently, toxic products build up in your bloodstream, your blood volume decreases and less oxygen and fewer nutrients are transported to your cells. Dehydration also results in your feeling weak and tired and can lead to over-eating as it disturbs appetite mechanisms and makes you think you are hungry even when you are not. The role of water in good health is almost completely ignored. The brain is seventy-five per cent water. This is why the quantity and quality of water you drink also affects how you think and feel. Thoughts and feelings become distorted when your body gets even mildly dehydrated. For mental clarity and emotional balance you need plenty of water. But if the water you drink is polluted by heavy metals or chemicals, the biochemical reactions on which clear thought and emotional balance depend will become polluted as well.

Liquid Energy

Drinking enough brings dynamic energy. Yet few of us drink enough. When Sir Edmund Hillary set out to conquer Everest he had a shrewd doctor named George Hunt on his ascent team. Hunt knew this precept well. He had studied the records of the recent failed attempt by the Swiss team and discovered that their climbers had drunk less than two glasses of water a day each. So he ordered special battery-operated snow-melting equipment and urged the British climbers to drink a minimum of twelve glasses of water each day of the climb to reduce their fatigue as they scaled the peaks.

Since then, research with athletes at Harvard University and Loma Linda University in the United States carried out to explore the relationship between water consumption and energy has demonstrated that drinking extra water reduces fatigue and stress and increases stamina and energy to a remarkable degree. During one of the Harvard studies, researcher G.C. Pitts set athletes walking at 5.6 k.p.h. (3^1/2 m.p.h.), allowing them to rest regularly, but not allowing them to drink extra water. They reached exhaustion after three and a half hours with temperatures of 102 degrees Fahrenheit. Under the same conditions, he allowed them to drink as much as they wanted. The same athletes lasted six hours before collapsing. In the thrd study, athletes were forced to drink more water than thirst dictated, in quantities the researchers calculated would replace what was being lost in perspiration. This time the athletes were able to continue indefinitely without fatigue or fever until finally, after running out of time, the researchers were forced to bring the experiment to a close. Few of us drink as much water as we need to remain in top form. Even if you pay attention to your thirst and quench it regularly, you are likely to replace only about a half to two-thirds of the water your body needs for optimal health.

Water Power

Water plays a major part in digesting your foods and absorbing nutrients thanks to enzymes which are themselves mostly water. If you fail to drink enough water between meals your mouth becomes low in saliva and digestion suffers. Water is also the medium through which wastes are eliminated from your body. Each time you exhale you release highly humidified air – about two big glasses' worth a day. Your kidneys and intestines eliminate another six or so glasses every twenty-four hours, while another two glasses' worth are released through the pores of your skin. This is on a cool day.

When it gets hot, when you are exercising, or when you are working hard, the usual ten glasses lost in this way can triple. On average, in a temperate climate – not sweating from exertion or heat – we need about 3.5 litres (6 pints) a day for optimal health although few of us consume as much a third of that amount. The important thing to remember is that thirst is not a reliable indication of how much water you need to drink. If you want to grow lean and stay healthy, you need to do as French women have done for decades. Keep a large bottle or two of pure, fresh, mineral water on your desk and make sure you consume your quota of this clear, delicious health-giving drink. Here's how to work out how many glasses of water you should drink a day:

> Divide your current weight in kilos by eight. Say you weigh 58 kilos (9st 11): 58 divided by eight equals 7.25 big glasses. Round the figure upwards to the next glass and there you have it: eight glasses a day. But remember, that is only a base calculation for a cool day. You will need a lot more during exercise, or on a hot day.

Provided you do not suffer from a kidney or liver disease, drinking eight big glasses or more of water a day not only helps you to lose weight and keep it off permanently, it improves the functioning of your whole body. There is another way in which drinking optimal quantities of water plays a central role in detoxifying the body for regeneration. It has to do with your kidneys.

The Regulators

The kidneys are responsible for recycling all the water in your body and for filtering out any wastes present before they can lower immunity, create fatigue, or make you feel hungry even though you have had enough to eat, and cause the kind of water retention which plagues so many who have gone on and off slimming diets for years. The filtering mechanism responsible for all this in the kidneys is made up of millions of microscopic bodies known as *glomeruli*. They identify waste products such as urea which need to be removed, as well as screening out other chemicals, unwanted metals and minerals and pouring back into the bloodstream the minerals you do need and regulating your body's acid–alkaline balance.

When some part of you needs more water, your kidneys make sure it arrives. For instance, when you are hot and sweating, a message is sent to the pituitary gland in the head telling it to release the anti-diuretic hormone, which in turn tells your kidneys to let more water be resorbed into the blood. Your urine at such times can become highly concentrated and a dark colour. But provided you replenish the water you are losing in sweat by drinking more, your kidneys will continue to function well and the appetite/thirst messages from your brain will not become confused. When your body's water level gets too low from not drinking enough, your kidneys cannot carry out their cleansing efficiently and the liver's role in detoxification becomes over-burdened. Water is the world's best natural diuretic. If your body tends to retain water, this is often because you don't drink enough, and it is holding on to what water there is. Once you do begin to drink enough, this tendency to waterlogging decreases and usually disappears completely. And, by the way, if you are worried about puckered thighs, the easiest way to help eliminate them is to drink more water. During a Miso Detox and Rebuild you need to drink plenty of water. Keep a 1.5-litre bottle on your desk or in your room and see that you drain it every day, regardless of whatever else you drink.

Clean and Clear

The quality of water you drink matters a lot too. If you can afford the best spring waters, buy them. If not, at least get yourself a good water filter and use it always, changing it regularly. Bottled waters differ tremendously. Some of those sold in plastic containers or glass bottles in the supermarket are nothing more than tap water which has been run through conditioning filters to remove the taste while doing nothing to improve the quality. The fact that the word 'spring' appears on the label doesn't mean a thing. It may simply be part of the brand name used to sell the product. Other bottled waters are excellent in taste and quality. Few countries except France do much to regulate standards for bottled water and what regulation there is is generally even poorer than that applied to tap water.

There are some twelve hundred registered springs in France. Several dozen of them supply bottled waters the quality of which has long been monitored and controlled by official government bodies. A few have been granted the title '*eau minerale naturelle*'. This means that they maintain a constant mineral content. It also means that they have a reputation for specific therapeutic properties. These waters should be safe from bacterial or chemical contamination and you can be sure they are not mixed with any foreign substance when they are bottled. Two of the best mineral waters are Volvic, an exceptionally pure still water from the Auvergne mountains in central France, and the sparkling Perrier which arrives in a carbonated form from a spring in Vergeze in Southern France. The Volvic spring is surrounded by 4400 hectares (11,000 acres) of countryside free from industry, intensive farming and other nearby sources of pollution. Volvic is lightly mineralised with a lot of character and a vibrant quality. Vittel is also good, as is Evian.

Get the Habit

It takes a bit of practice to make sure you get your water quota each day, but soon it will become second nature. Start by drinking two glasses of water first thing in the morning when you get up, either neat or with a twist of lemon or lime. You can heat the water if you like. This helps with elimination. Then drink two or three glasses between breakfast and lunch and another two or three between lunch and dinner.

When you exercise or when it is hot, remember to drink more. Getting the water habit will quench your appetite, improve your body's ability to eliminate wastes, heighten your energy levels, improve the look of your skin and help your metabolic processes to function at peak. You will be amazed to discover just how potent are its gifts.

Here is an action plan for water during the Miso Detox and Rebuild which is also excellent to follow afterwards:

- Divide your weight in kilos by eight, then round up to the next glass to discover how many large glasses of water to drink each day.
- Drink two glasses of mineral or filtered water on rising and complete your daily quota by drinking further glasses between meals.
- Keep a bottle or two of mineral water by you during the day as an easy measure of the quantity you need to drink to get your daily quota.
- Sit back and watch your energy increase.

Rest and Repair

During a Miso Detox and Rebuild it is also important to get plenty of rest. You will need more than usual, for much of your body's energy will be involved in deep cleansing itself. Take a nap in the middle of the day whenever you can and spend more time in bed at night reading or listening to music, making love or doing anything else that gives you pleasure. It can also be helpful to take long walks, get plenty of gentle exercise, and brush your skin before you bath or shower using a dry, natural bristle brush.

Almost a third of the body's waste products are eliminated through the skin. Skin brushing is a gentle yet powerful way to stimulate lymphatic drainage and encourage the elimination of wastes. Spend five minutes a day, before your bath, brushing your skin all over with a dry, natural bristle brush. Begin at the tips of your shoulders and cover your whole body (except the head) with long smooth strokes, going downwards over the shoulders, arms and trunk, then upwards over the feet, legs and hips. You need only go over your skin once for it to work. The most amazing quantity of rubbish can come out of skin that is brushed regularly. Check for yourself by rubbing a damp flannel over your freshly scrubbed body. Hang up the flannel and use it to repeat the process for a few days. You will find the flannel soon smells of the waste products that have come directly through the skin's surface. Be grateful they are now outside your body and no longer inside!

Cleansing Reactions

When you replace the foods you are accustomed to eat with cleansing and regenerating foods, your body starts throwing off wastes with great abandon. This can lead to a few uncomfortable symptoms and it is as well to be prepared for them. You may find your tongue and teeth take on a film that tastes unpleasant, for instance. You may have a headache (especially if you have been a heavy coffee drinker). You may feel a little under the weather, even a bit nauseous. A very few people run a mild fever in the first couple of days. Any of these symptoms – and they by no means occur in every case – are simply a sign that the detox is working. Be pleased. These cleansing reactions quickly pass.

Taking an Epsom salts bath can help to relieve feelings of discomfort or irritability. Pour two cups of household grade Epsom salts (available from your local chemist) into a blood-heat bath. Immerse yourself for twenty to thirty minutes, topping up with warm water to maintain a comfortable temperature. If you have a headache, simply go and lie down in a quiet, dark room if you can. Sipping a cup of peppermint tea or green tea will also help. If you find you have difficulty getting to sleep, try quietly sipping a cup of camomile tea before bed, or take tincture of valerian or passionflower (see pages 125–126).

The Psychic Detox

During a detox, all sorts of anxieties, guilt and insecurities that have been locked inside the rubbish our bodies have been carrying around suddenly seem to come to the surface. They will be flushed away along with the toxins. It can also be an excellent time to explore meditation or practise a deep relaxation exercise once or twice a day, or to begin recording your dreams. The whole process of deep-cleansing the body – breaking out of habits of living which do not support health and energy at the highest levels – is but one part of cleansing your whole self, including mind, emotions and spirit. It can open up new vistas and help you to see your whole life in new ways; it is often useful to record these things, since they may be very different from the way we habitually look at our lives. I first discovered this when, under the supervision of a health practitioner, I did my first fast at the age of twenty-eight and found the clarity I needed to work out which direction in life to take.

As stored wastes are eliminated from your body, your skin will take on a new glow and translucence. Lines on your face will be softened and your eyes will become clear and bright. In addition, your mind will become clearer so that thinking is easier. Many writers and artists use detoxification regimes before beginning a new project because they can heighten creativity. It is no accident that throughout history saints and philosophers have turned to abstinence – another way to cleanse body and psyche – as a way of increasing spiritual awareness and improving mental clarity. Following this kind of regime for a week or several weeks can create a bridge between an existence in which you have not cared for yourself well and a whole new way of living. It is a mid-life ritual that can bring not just regeneration on a physical level, but the resurrection of your self-esteem as you learn to value and protect your own health and wellbeing.

Step Four
Level Up

THE DECISIONS you make about how and what you eat from the age of thirty-five onwards not only largely determine the kind of menopause you will have and how protected you are from osteoporosis, they also determine how slowly or rapidly your body ages, how good you look and feel as the years pass and how much energy you have. Life feeds upon life. The secret to eating for a natural menopause is what Step Four is all about. It means making use of wholesome foods radiant with life that increase mental and physical energy and prevent premature ageing while restoring hormonal order.

The theory is simple; the practice is more complicated. The first thing you need to do is to forsake once and for all convenience foods with their hidden fat and sugar. It is important to be well informed about fats too, since nothing can disrupt a woman's hormonal system like processed fats in foods, and these junk fats are just about everywhere. Instead, opt for a life-generating way of eating based on simple wholesome foods grown on healthy soils. Incorporate foods rich in phyto-hormones – natural hormones that perfectly fit your own receptor sites and prevent damage by oestrogen mimics – found in raw foods, concentrated green foods like spirulina and chlorella, and naturally fermented foods from the Orient such as miso. Learn the ropes and you will create a way of eating that naturally rebalances hormones and restores vibrant health.

Loaded with Energy

Carbohydrates are your body's main source of energy for all its functions. However, just any old carbohydrate won't do.

Only complex carbohydrates – fruits and vegetables, unre-
fined grains, sea plants and legumes – provide steady lasting
energy throughout the day. One of the major problems of
eating processed foods full of simple carbohydrates like white
flour and sugar is that they bring about a progressive decline
in your body's ability to process sugar. Unlike natural
foods full of protective fibre, refined and processed foods are
highly concentrated. Fibre is no longer present to dilute their
concentration and to slow down the rate at which the simple
starches and sugars they contain are absorbed into your
bloodstream. Such foods are far more calorie-dense. If you
eat them year after year, they begin to overwhelm the body –
especially the pancreas – causing blood sugar problems and
mood and energy swings that wreak havoc with your health.
Don't be misled by the nonsense that is written on the
packaging of foods you buy, either. Read the ingredients
carefully and watch for hidden sugars: *glucose, sorbitol, invert
sugar, corn syrup, maltodextrin, dextrose, barley syrup, malt
sugar*. These are just alternative names for sugar. Even many
products which claim to be sugar-free contain one or more of
them.

Caffeine – found in coffee, tea and many soft drinks – gives
you a quick lift and the illusion of energy only to let you crash
down a couple of hours later. Then you may be inclined to
reach for more – or for a sticky bun or chocolate – just to keep
going. Tea contains a surprising 100 milligrams of caffeine per
cup to coffee's 120 milligrams. Coffee also makes the blood
more acid, which in turn draws calcium from your bones to
try to re-establish a healthy acid–alkaline balance. Drinking
coffee is one of the worst things you can do if you want to
prevent osteoporosis. Many colas, squashes and soft drinks
contain caffeine. And they are far too high in sugar. A regular
can of cola contains seven teaspoons of sugar – about
40 grams (1$^{1}/_{2}$ oz). As for the 'diet' varieties, they are an even
more unpleasant chemical cocktail full of excess phosphorous
and additives which only pollute your body and further
contribute to calcium loss from bones. Stay away from them.

All Fats Are Not Equal

Each of us in the West consumes about 175 grams (6 oz) of fat a day. That makes a horrifying 63 kilograms (138 lb) of fat a year. Between forty and fifty per cent of our food calories come from fat. For good long-term health you need to reduce your fat intake down to fifteen to twenty-five per cent of the calories you eat. Look at the packaging on foods such as milk, cheese, biscuits and bread, and read the list of proteins, carbohydrates and fats they contain, and the calories per serving. You can make some quick calculations to tell you what percentage of the calories in the food are fat calories. Here's how to work it out:

> Say a packet of biscuits contains 145 calories per 100-gram serving, made up of 4 grams of protein, 19 grams of carbohydrate, and 7 grams of fat. Multiply the amount of fat by ten (rounded up from fat being nine calories per gram), i.e. add a zero to the number of grams of fat per serving to give you how many of the calories per serving are in the form of fat. Then compare this figure with the total calories. In this case it would be 7 x 10 = 70 calories of fat in each 145 calories. Divide 70 by 145 and you get 0.48. This tells you the biscuits are about forty-eight per cent fat. As this is way above the limit of twenty-five per cent for optimal health, reject the packet.

But this is not the only thing you need to know about fat. You also need to take great care to make sure that the fat calories you do eat are the right kind. For the kind of fats you eat largely determines the hormonal health of your body.

The Good Guys and the Bad Guys

All fats and oils in our foods are made out of fatty acids, molecules that have a fat part and an acid part. Saturated fats – found in meat, dairy products like cheese, ice-cream, milk, and the tropical oils like palm kernel oil and coconut – are stable, inactive and virtually inert in your body. Their major *raison d'être* is to provide calories in a concentrated form which can later be burned as energy. Eat too many foods full of saturated fats and they do their best to lay themselves down as fat stores. You will get as much saturated fat as you need from your food without ever giving it a second thought.

Unsaturated fats are different. They come in two forms: mono-unsaturates like olive oil, and poly-unsaturates, found in corn, sunflower seeds, peanuts and many other foods. They can more readily take part in important biochemical changes in your body that produce energy, create hormones, and help burn stored body fats. The right unsaturated fats are essential to a woman's hormonal health all through her reproductive life and beyond. But a lot of hokum about unsaturated fats is spread about by sellers of margarine and producers of processed junk foods.

Natural, unadulterated, unsaturated fats come in a chemical configuration known as a *cis* form. This is the only form a woman's body can use for anything except pumping up her fat stores. Cis fatty acids are destroyed by the modern processing that turns out the golden oils stacked on the shelves of our supermarkets, oils with which the mass-produced foods we eat today are riddled. Cis fatty acids – the good guys – are rather like 'gloves' that fit perfectly onto the 'hands' of the molecular fat receptors in your body. Trans fatty acids are bad guys. They not only don't properly fit into your body's metabolic machinery, they can even block fat receptor sites and interfere with your ability to produce important hormones, thus causing PMS and menopausal miseries. Since trans fatty acids don't occur in nature, our bodies have never developed any mechanisms for making use of them. They treat them as foreign invaders and do their best to protect us from them by trying to store them away, laying them down as fat, even in our arteries.

Bare Essentials

Your body can make all the fat it needs for daily metabolic processes except for two *essential fatty acids*. These are found naturally in fresh foods – in seeds and nuts, in vegetables and fish – and even in wild meat such as game. For optimum health you need no more than two to four tablespoons of these essential fatty acids a day, yet despite our high fat intake in the West, they can be as hard to find in modern convenience foods as the proverbial hen's teeth. These two unsaturates help you to burn body fat and build energy; they also help your body to manufacture important hormones. They are called essential fatty acids because that is exactly what they are: essential to human life and health. The problem with linoleic and linolenic acids – both of which are unsaturated fats – is that the chemical reactivity which gives them their health-giving power also makes them highly unstable, so they spoil easily. Natural foods that contain them, such as grains and seeds, will turn rancid in contact with air because unsaturated fats oxidise rapidly, although their rancidity may not be noticeable by taste or smell. A good diet based on wholesome foods, with a good proportion of fresh, raw fruits and vegetables, will give you plenty of essential fatty acids. One of the best ways of getting extra quantities of essential fatty acids is to buy vacuum-packed flax seeds, pulverise them and sprinkle a dessertspoonful or two on your cereals or salads every day. Using Udo's Choice, an oil blend in perfect balance of basic essential fatty acids, is even better (see Resources).

Cry Wild

Raw foods do wonderful things for women. Human evolution is a slow process. For hundreds of generations our ancestors lived on wild foods gathered and eaten raw. Our genes appear to be specially adapted to dealing with raw foods. Incorporating a good percentage of live foods – fresh vegetables, raw seeds and nuts, fresh sprouted grains and seeds – in your diet can help to rebalance hormones, stabilise moods, clear and rejuvenate skin, shed excess fat and transform your whole outlook on life. Eat fifty per cent of your foods raw and choose the rest from wholesome natural products such as grains and pulses, sea plants, cooked vegetables, fresh locally grown fruits and naturally produced soya products such as miso and tofu, and you will probably notice a dramatic improvement in how you look and feel and function within the first couple of weeks. But it will be several weeks before the burden of toxicity which you have been carrying has fully cleared, and it will probably be a few months before even deeper benefits begin to show themselves. So be patient. Your body has a magnificent ability to heal itself, but this doesn't happen overnight.

Ideally the foods you eat on a high-raw diet should be chosen from fresh, organically grown vegetables and fruits, for these foods offer the highest complement of substances of nutritional value. But for me, as for most people, this is just not possible. I grow my own herbs and a few fruits and vegetables in my garden in the country, but half of the time I live in a flat in the city and there I have little access to anything which has been organically grown. Making at least one meal a day a big raw salad of sprouted seeds and grains and all sorts of raw vegetables – from raw beetroot to raw herbs, carrots, cauliflower, whatever is in season – solves, at least in part, the dilemma about organically grown foods because, since you've grown the sprouts yourself, you know that they haven't been subjected to any chemical treatments, and because you have used (or should have used) spring water to grow them, they will not contain any undesirable minerals or other chemicals. Your salad is an excellent source of top quality protein, essential fatty acids, and natural sugars. When seeds are sprouted the starch they contain begins to be broken down and turned into natural sugars which are easy to assimilate and provide energy to heighten your mood. Finally, and probably most important of all, remember that home-grown sprouts are brimming with life energy. This life energy – the very basis of the power which can transform your health, your shape, your energy and your appearance, is as yet little understood; it is only beginning to be measured, using sensitive instruments.

Seed Journey

Sprouted seeds and grains, which you can easily grow on your kitchen window sill or in your airing cupboard (see pages 70–72), are the richest known source of naturally occurring vitamins. They are also the most prolific of all foods: a mere teaspoonful of alfalfa seeds will produce over 200 grams (8oz) of sprouts.; just 125 grams (4^1/2 oz) of mung seeds will produce a kilo (2^1/2 lb) of bean sprouts. Sprouts come in all shapes and colours, from the tiny curlicue forms of green alfalfa to the round yellow spheres of chickpeas. Easy seeds/grains/pulses for sprouting include: alfalfa, mung beans, adzuki (aduki) beans, wheat, barley, fenugreek, lentils, mustard, oats, pumpkin, sesame, soya beans and sunflower. When a seed sprouts, enzymes which have been dormant in it spring into action, breaking down stored starch and turning it into simple natural sugars and splitting long-chain proteins into amino acids. What this means is that the process of sprouting turns these seeds into foods which are very easily digested. They have many times the nutritional goodness of the seeds from which they have grown. Gram for gram, they provide more nutrients than any other natural food.

In an age when most vegetables and fruits are grown on artificially fertilised soils and treated with hormones, fungicides, insecticides, preservatives and all manner of other chemicals, the home-grown-in-a-jar sprout emerges as a pristine blessing – fresh, unpolluted and ready to eat in salads or sandwiches. Sprouts are a wonderful health food for any family concerned about the rising cost of food and the falling nutritional value of the average diet, for they are the cheapest form of natural food around. Different sprouts mixed together will support life all on their own. While I would never suggest that anybody live on sprouts alone, I think they are an ideal addition to the table – particularly if the budget is tight.

Phyto-Hormone Plant Power

To help you to reap the rewards of a natural menopause, go for foods high in phyto-hormones – compounds in plants whose molecular structure is akin to the body's own hormones. Unlike dangerous xenoestrogens, plant hormones are weak in their actions. They 'fit' into a woman's metabolism. Your body recognises them and knows how to use them. When weak oestrogens from plants bind with oestrogen receptor sites in the body, they help to protect the body from the negative effects of xenoestrogens and the body's own stronger oestrogens. They allow the body to readjust its own hormonal balance naturally. This is why a diet high in soya bean products such as tofu plays such an important part in protecting Japanese women from hormone-related diseases. Vitamins, minerals and phyto-hormones in fresh foods eaten as close as possible to the state in which they come out of the ground – or carefully and naturally fermented, as they are in Japan – can supply enough phyto-hormones to mitigate most of the symptoms that plague women in industrialised countries, from fibrocystic breast disease, PMS and hot flushes to osteoporosis.

Some of the best hormone-rich foods to add to your diet, both as protection against health problems and for the sake of overall vitality, are the green foods: spirulina, chlorella, the seaweeds, sprouted alfalfa and green barley. Eating some of the green foods every day can slowly, over a period of several months, help to replenish what may have been lost for many years. This is something that is very difficult to achieve in any other way, for in order for minerals to be well assimilated they need to be highly bio-available – your body needs to be able to make use of them easily. Most vitamin and mineral supplements are not bio-available. Seaweeds, chlorella, spirulina and green barley are also wonderful cleansing foods, helping to detoxify the body of excess oestrogens as well as other pollutants, and they are excellent energy enhancers. You can buy powdered green foods such as spirulina, green barley and chlorella and mix a tablespoon of them into a glass of juice. Sprinkle seaweeds liberally on your salads. The natural tendency of the human body is to strengthen and heal itself, and it relishes the nutritional elements that can help it to do so. Green foods have much to offer.

Natural Protection

So many fresh foods are rich in plant hormones. Include them often in your meals. The fresher they are the better: yams, peas, papayas, bananas, cucumbers, raw nuts, bee pollen, sprouted seeds and grains, and the herbs liquorice root, alfalfa, red clover, sage, sarsaparilla and sassafras. Raw fruits and vegetables, green vegetable juices, figs and garlic, dates, avocados, grapes, apples, seaweed, wheat germ and chlorella can all be helpful in countering menopausal and menstrual problems. Grapes, cherries, citrus fruits and red clover are excellent sources of the bioflavonoids, which also have weak oestrogenic activity and have been shown to be useful in countering hot flushes and mood swings and in helping to prevent heavy, irregular menstrual flow. Plant foods high in phyto-hormones are good insurance against cancer too since they help to prevent oestrogen-dominance in the body. The fibre found in plants is protective against oestrogen-dominance and cancer via another mechanism. Breast cancer is highly related to oestrogen levels as well as to over-consumption of meat and fat. Women on a vegetarian diet high in fibre excrete a much higher level of oestrogen than other women and have much lower levels of the hormone in the blood. In Britain and the United States the use of milk products has also been correlated with breast cancer. Sea plants and green vegetables, spirulina and chlorella are far better sources of calcium than cheese and milk. Some of the best natural hormone foods of all are the soya-based foods from the Orient, together with naturally fermented foods – often of Japanese origin. Include plenty of them in your diet – tofu, miso, tamari, soya flour and soya milk.

Change of Life

Making changes in the way you eat means making changes in how you cook and shop. You may find your larder stocked with a whole new set of ingredients – particularly if until now you have been living on convenience foods or meat and two veg. The foods which you will use for most of the recipes in this book are not only good for you, they are delicious: grains and legumes, nuts and seeds, fruits, vegetables and herbs. They can be very expensive or, if you shop around, very cheap. I buy many of my fruits in crates from a wholesaler at less than half the price I would pay at the greengrocer's. You can pay high prices for nuts, seeds, grains and pulses in some health food stores where they come in tiny packages (and are often not very fresh). But beans, legumes, nuts and seeds can also be bought cheaply in good supermarkets or in bulk at reasonable cost from many of the new whole-food emporiums which are beginning to appear everywhere. Obviously the more you buy at one time the cheaper they are. Be sure to refrigerate nuts after purchase to keep their oils from going rancid. And if ever you find, on returning home, that something you have bought is not absolutely fresh, take it back and complain. That is the best way to protect yourself while improving the quality of what is being sold into the bargain. Here is a brief guide to stocking a larder with life-generating foods, to give you some idea of just how much variety you have to choose from:

Fruits

Not only are fruits some of the most delicious natural foods available, they also have remarkable properties for spring-cleaning the body and are excellent biochemical antidotes to the stress that ages. Fruit contains very little protein but it is very high in potassium, a mineral which needs to be balanced with sodium for perfect health in the body. Most people in the West eat far too much sodium in the form of table salt, in addition to an excess of protein (which leaches important minerals from the bones and tissues), so eating good quantities of fruit can help to re-balance the body, improve its functioning and increase energy. Because fruits are naturally sweet, and because we are born with an innate liking for sweet things, a dessert of fresh fruit after a meal can be tremendously satisfying to the palate. And there is such a variety of beautiful textures, colours and tastes to choose from – from the sensuous softness of persimmons and the super-sweetness of fresh figs, to the exhilarating crunch of the finest English apple.

Vegetables

The best vegetables are those you grow yourself organically. If you are lucky enough to have a garden – even a small one – save all your leftovers and turn them into compost for fertiliser. Even in winter you can grow some delicious salads and root vegetables in a greenhouse or under cloches. The quality of organic produce is far superior to chemically fertilised fruits and vegetables – not to mention all the vitamins which are lost when foods are picked, stored, shipped and left sitting on shop shelves. In the summer I go to the garden to pick my vegetables and fifteen minutes later they are gracing the dinner table. That is the best way to preserve their nutritional value as well as to experience the fullness of their flavour. If you live in a flat without a garden you can sprout fresh seeds and grains in jars or trays on your windowsill (see page 67). Scrubbing vegetables is better than peeling them, because many of the valuable vitamins and minerals are stored directly beneath their skins. Never soak vegetables for long periods. Wash them briefly under running water to prevent water-soluble vitamins leaching out of them. Always keep vegetables as cool as possible (even carrots and turnips are best kept in the fridge) and use them as soon as you can. Be demanding when you shop: choose your own cauliflower and make sure it is a good one. Don't be intimidated by pushy greengrocers who want to fob you off with the leftovers before they bring in their new stock. Demand the best and you will get it. Your palate and your health will be grateful to you.

Grains

When you eat a good portion of grain foods, you are likely to find that your general disposition improves, you feel calm, and have energy that lasts and lasts. Grains, like legumes, need special handling. They should not be eaten raw. This is why many of the packaged mueslis cause digestive upset in many people. It is only by cooking them (or by sprouting or soaking them, even by lightly toasting them) that you break the chemical bonds, turning hard-to-digest starches into more easily digested sugars. The other important thing to remember about grains is that it is best to get as wide a variety as possible, so if you have oat porridge at breakfast, at lunch you might choose whole rye bread, a bulgur wheat salad or brown rice. The more variety the better, since each grain has a different balance of essential minerals and micronutrients. Here is a quick guide to cooking them:

Guide to Cooking Grains

Grain (1 cup)	Water (cups)	Cooking time	Yield (cups)
Barley – whole	4–5	2–3 hours	$3^{1}/_{2}$
Barley – flakes	3	45–60 minutes	3
Brown rice	2–$2^{1}/_{2}$	1 hour	3
Buckwheat	2	20 minutes	$2^{1}/_{2}$
Bulgar wheat	2	15–20 minutes	$2^{1}/_{2}$
Couscous	1	15 minutes	$2^{3}/_{4}$
Millet	$2^{1}/_{2}$–3	45–60 minutes	$3^{1}/_{2}$
Oats – whole groats	5	2–3 hours	$2^{1}/_{2}$
Polenta	5	45–60 minutes	$3^{1}/_{2}$
Rye	5	2–3 hours	2
Quinoa	2	20 minutes	$2^{1}/_{2}$
Wild rice	3	1–$1^{1}/_{2}$ hours	$3^{1}/_{2}$
Wheat – whole grain	5	2–3 hours	$2^{1}/_{2}$
Wheat flakes	2	45–60 minutes	3

Oils

It is wise not to use oils, except for Udo's Choice, flaxseed oil and extra virgin olive oil on your salads or, in tiny amounts, for wok frying. The oil found in flaxseed or linseed is an almost perfect balance of linoleic and linolenic acid, both the omega 6 and omega 3 essential fatty acids. I often simply grind flaxseed in a coffee grinder and then put it into a tightly covered jar and store it in the refrigerator. I then use two to four dessertspoons a day sprinkled over salads. It is important to go for the very best vacuum-packed linseeds, however, in order to make sure that the precious fatty acids which they contain are protected from rancidity (see Resources). It is as easy as that to make sure you get all the essential fatty acids you need. Steer clear of junk fats and processed oils; your body will do the rest.

Nuts

Fresh nuts are a good source of essential fatty acids when used in small quantities. However, the rancid oils in old nuts are harmful to the stomach. If nuts are fresh and whole (unbroken) you can buy a kilo or so at a time and, provided they are kept in an airtight container in a cool, dry place – ideally in the fridge – they will keep for a few months. You can even freeze them to keep them longer. It is a good idea to buy a few different kinds of nuts to give you plenty of variety in your recipes. Choose from: almonds, brazils, cashews, coconut (fresh or desiccated), hazels, macadamia nuts, pecans, pine kernels, pistachios, tiger nuts and walnuts.

Legumes

Nutritious, economical and delicious when well prepared, beans and pulses are rich in complex carbohydrates, protein, and fibre as well as minerals and essential fatty acids. They need careful preparation and cooking in order to avoid digestive upset, and should never be eaten raw. Legumes should first be washed and cleaned of any small pieces of stone or spoilt food. Then all except lentils, split peas and mung beans should be soaked for at least four to six hours, preferably overnight, before cooking. The soak water should then be thrown away and fresh water should be added. There are two ways to minimise digestive upset when cooking legumes; I use both of them. After soaking and rinsing, put your beans in the freezer overnight and cook them the next day. The second is after soaking, throw the soak water away, boil up the beans in fresh water for twenty minutes, throw the boil water away and rinse the beans, then add fresh water plus any vegetables, herbs and seasonings you are using, and cook them in a covered saucepan. Bring the beans to the boil, then reduce the heat and simmer them until they grow tender. I bring the beans to the boil and put them in a slow cooker or the bottom of my Aga oven and forget about them for six to eight hours. There are so many wonderful dishes you can make with legumes that you could fill ten cookery books with recipes. I like to use them to make thick soups and casseroles.

Beans and Pulses

Legumes (1 cup)	Soak	Water (cups)	Cooking time (hours)	Yield (cups)
Adzuki	Yes	4	3	2
Baby lima	Yes	3	2	$1^3/4$
Black beans	Yes	5	2	2
Cassoulet	Yes	4	$3^1/2$	2
Chickpeas	Yes	4	$3^1/2$	$2^1/2$
Kidney	Yes	3	$1^1/2$	2
Lentils	No	4	1	$2^1/4$
Lima	Yes	5	2	$1^1/4$
Mung	No	$2^1/2$	$1^1/2$	2
Navy	Yes	3	$2^1/2$	2
Pinto	Yes	3	$2^1/2$	2
Red	Yes	3	$3^1/2$	2
Split peas	No	3	1	$2^1/4$

They are also great cooked and used cold the next day as a base for a salad. I soak lima beans, black-eyed beans, kidney beans, and a mixture of beans, pour the soak water away, rinse the beans, then store them frozen in bags so that I can pull them out whenever I need them to make a casserole or a soup. The chart on page 69 will give you some guidelines to the cooking of legumes.

Sprouts

Seeds and grains are latent powerhouses of nutritional goodness and life energy. Add water to germinate them, let them grow for a few days in your kitchen and you will harvest delicious, inexpensive fresh foods of quite phenomenal health-enhancing value. The vitamin content of seeds increases dramatically when they germinate. The vitamin C content in soya beans multiplies five times within three days of germination – a mere tablespoon of soya bean sprouts contains half the recommended daily adult requirements of this vitamin. The vitamin B_2 in an oat grain rises by 1300 per cent almost as soon as the seed sprouts, and by the time tiny leaves have formed, it has risen by 2000 per cent. Some sprouted seeds and grains are believed to have anti-cancer properties, which is why they form an important part of the natural methods of treating the disease. Another attractive thing about sprouts is their price. The basic seeds and grains are cheap and readily available in supermarkets and health-food stores – chickpeas, brown lentils, mung beans, wheat grains, etc. And since you sprout them yourself with nothing but clean water, they are an easily accessible source of organically grown fresh vegetables, even for city dwellers.

DIY Sprouting

When you discover how economical and easy it is to grow sprouts you will want to have some on the go all the time. Once germinated, sprouts can be kept in polythene bags in the fridge for up to a week – just long enough to grow a new batch ready for eating. Most people grow sprouts in glass jars covered with nylon mesh held in place with an elastic band around the neck, but I have discovered an even simpler method; it allows you to grow many more sprouts and avoids the problem of seeds rotting, due to insufficient drainage, which can happen with the jar method.

You will need the following:

seeds (e.g. mung beans)
seed trays with drainage holes – from gardening shops and
    nurseries
a jar or bowl to soak seeds in overnight
a plant atomiser – from gardening or hardware shops
a sieve
nylon mesh – from gardening shops.

1. Place two handfuls of seeds or beans in a jar or bowl and cover with plenty of water. Leave to soak overnight.

2. Pour the seeds into a sieve and rinse well with water. Remove any dead or broken seeds or pieces of debris.

3. Line a seed tray with nylon mesh (this helps the seeds to drain better) and pour in the soaked seeds.

4. Place in a warm, dark place (such as the airing cupboard) for fast growth.

5. Spray the seeds twice a day with fresh water using an atomiser and stir them gently with your hand in order to aerate them.

6. After about three days, place the seeds in sunlight for several hours to develop the chlorophyll (green) in them.

7. Rinse the seeds in a sieve, drain well and put in a polythene bag in the fridge to use in salads, wok-fries, etc.

There are many different seeds you can sprout, each with its own particular flavour and texture. Use the following chart as a guide.

Sprouting

Seeds	Soak time	To Yield 1 litre	Ready to eat in	Length of shoot	Growing tips and notes
Alfalfa	6–8 hours	3–4 tbsp	5–6 days	3.5 cm (1¹/₂ in)	Rich in organic vitamins and minerals and natural oestrogens.
Fenugreek	6–8 hours	¹/₂ cup	3–4 days	1 cm (¹/₂ in)	Have quite a strong 'curry' taste. Good for ridding the body of toxins.
Adzuki beans	10–15 hours	1¹/₂ cups	3–5 days	2.5–3.5 cm (1–1¹/₂ in)	Have a nutty flavour. Especially good for the kidneys.
Chickpeas	10–15 hours	2 cups	3–4 days	2.5 cm (1 in)	May need to soak for eighteen hours to swell to their full size. Replace the water during this time.
Lentils	10–15 hours	1 cup	3–5 days	0.5–2.5cm (¹/₄–1 in)	Try all different kinds of lentils. They are good eaten young or up to six days old.
Mung beans	10–15 hours	1 cup	3–5 days	1–5 cm (¹/₂–2¹/₂ in)	Soak at least fifteen hours. Keep in the dark for a sweet sprout.
Sunflower seeds	10–15 hours	4 cups	1–2 days	Same length as seed	Sprout them for just one day. They bruise easily so handle carefully.
Wheat	12–15 hours	2 cups	2–3 days	Same length as grain	An excellent source of the B vitamins. The soak water can be drunk straight or added to soups and vegetable juices.

Sea Vegetables

If you have never used the sea vegetables for cooking, this is an ideal time to begin. Not only are they delicious, imparting a wonderful, spicy flavour to soups and salads, they are the richest natural source of organic mineral salts, particularly of iodine. Iodine is the mineral needed by the thyroid gland. As this gland is largely responsible for the body's metabolic rate, iodine is very important to a woman's energy. Get to know some of the sea vegetables and start to make use of them. Your body, and especially your nails and hair, will be strengthened by the full range of minerals and trace elements they contain, such as selenium, calcium, iodine, boron, potassium, magnesium and iron which are not always found in great quantities in our ordinary garden vegetables. I like to use powdered kelp as a seasoning. It adds both flavour and minerals to salad dressings, salads, soups and so forth. I am also very fond of nori seaweed, which comes in long, thin sheets or tiny flakes. It is a delicious snack food which you can eat along with a salad or at the beginning of the meal; it has a beautiful, crisp flavour. I often toast it very, very quickly by putting it under a grill for no more than ten or fifteen seconds. It is also delicious raw. You can use nori to wrap around everything from a sprout salad to cooked grains in order to make little pieces of vegetarian sushi. It's often a good idea to soak some of the other sea vegetables such as dulse, arame and hiziki for a few minutes in enough tepid water to cover. This softens them so that they can be easily chopped and put into salads or added to soups. Sea vegetables are available in health-food stores and in oriental food shops. Recommended ones are: arame, dulse, hiziki, kelp, kombu, laver bread, nori, wakami, and mixed sea salad.

Tofu

Its other name is bean curd. This white, bland soft food made from soya beans is easy to digest, high in protein, low in calories and fat, cheap, and you can use it for just about anything. It will absorb whatever flavour you soak it in. When you cook it, it becomes firmer. You can mix it with herbs, use it to make sauces, low-fat mayonnaise, dips for vegetables, pizza toppings and stir fries. You can even substitute it for cheese in some of your favourite recipes; it won't melt under the grill, however. Buy tofu in the supermarket, health-food store or oriental food shop and keep it sitting in water in the fridge so that it doesn't dry out. As with any product made from soya beans, make sure the soya has not been genetically modified. Always choose organic soya products.

Miso

A fermented soya bean paste which is rich in digestive enzymes and high in protein, miso can be used for seasoning soups and sauces, or for making a wholesome broth. It is also a delicious addition to dips for crudités and salad dressings.

Tamari

This is a type of soya sauce made from fermented soya beans, but unlike soya sauce it contains no wheat, although it does contain sea salt and should therefore be used in moderation. It is good for giving a 'Chinese' taste to dishes as well as a rich flavour to bland dressings or sauces.

Soya Flour

Made from cooked, ground soya beans, soya flour is sometimes added to grain-based flours to increase their protein content. It can be used to make soya milk and soya cheese.

Soya Milk

Made from cooked, ground, and strained soya beans, this is often used for bottle-fed infants who are allergic to cow's milk. I use it as a substitute for milk on cereals and in recipes. Be careful when you buy it, as ready-made varieties are often packed in aluminium-lined cartons and it is best to avoid aluminium.

Seven Days of Supermeals

For energy that lasts, breakfast like a king, lunch like a prince and sup like a pauper, as the old adage recommends. For example, breakfast would be a bowl of miso broth or a grain dish, e.g. porridge with one or two pieces of fruit, whole-grain toast (wheat-free, ideally) with a fruit or nut spread. Lunch would become your main meal, consisting of a main course plus some vegetables – crudités, salads or sprouted seeds and grains, plus a yellow and green vegetable if not already incorporated – and whole-grain bread (again, wheat-free) and a fruit spread. Supper would be a light meal consisting of a fruit dish or perhaps a light soup.

Monday

Main meal   100 per cent corn pasta with garlic olive oil and steamed vegetables. A large salad made with shredded fresh raw carrots and tangerine sections dressed with orange juice, curry powder and chopped parsley. Follow with baked bananas made using organic brown rice syrup, a dash of rum and a squeeze of lemon juice.

Light meal   A salad of raw vegetables arranged in segments: grated carrots, red or yellow peppers, half an avocado, radish slices, a handful of Chinese bean sprouts, a few slices of cucumber, a grated raw beetroot or white radish and some mustard and cress. Dress with Tofu Vinaigrette: $3/4$ cup tofu, 3 tbsp rice wine vinegar or cider vinegar, the juice of 2 lemons, 1 tbsp Dijon mustard, 1 clove of garlic, crushed, salt and fresh herbs. Put in blender and process. The dressing will keep for a few days in the fridge.

Tuesday

Main meal   Carrot soup with orange and fresh ginger made from: $1/2$ cup chopped green onions, 1 cup orange juice, 1 cup water, 2 cups diced carrots, 2 tsp chopped fresh ginger, 2 tbsp low-salt vegetable bouillon (to taste), freshly ground pepper and 1 tsp of coriander. Boil the carrots until tender, then add the orange juice and bouillon powder. Reheat and serve along with slices of organic tofu which have been spread with miso and grilled. Serve with a selection of steamed vegetables. Follow with raw pineapple slices dusted with shredded coconut.

Light meal   A jacket potato stuffed with sprouted seeds or grains and Tofu Dip made from: 1 cup tofu, juice of 1 lemon, 1 tsp whole-grain mustard, 1 tbsp low-salt vegetable bouillon powder, a few leaves of fresh basil or some chopped parsley. Combine well in a food processor. This will keep for several days in the fridge.

Wednesday

Main meal   Grilled fresh mackerel with garlic and lemon juice served with a selection of steamed vegetables, or Split Pea Soup made from: 1 cup dried split peas (soaked overnight), 1 onion, 2 medium carrots, 2 sticks celery, 1 litre (1 3/4 pints) spring water, 1 tbsp low-salt vegetable bouillon powder, 2 tbsp chopped fresh herbs. Put the peas, vegetables and water into a pot, boil and simmer for 1 1/2 hours until the peas are tender. Add the vegetable bouillon and fresh herbs 5 minutes before serving. If you want a smooth soup, pour it into a food processor and blend. Serve with a salad of fresh young spinach leaves and sliced white mushrooms dressed with lemon and olive oil and sprinkled with toasted sunflower seeds. Follow with Orange Sorbet made from: 8 oranges (skin and seeds removed) pulped in a processor. Add a tiny amount of honey to sweeten and some nutmeg, ginger or fresh mint. Pour the mixture into ice-cube trays or a plastic container and freeze. Remove from the freezer and leave to thaw slightly for about ten minutes. Blend the mixture again immediately before serving.

Light meal   100 per cent buckwheat soba noodles in a bowl of miso broth. To cook the noodles, bring a big pot of water to the boil and add the noodles slowly so the water continues to boil. When it begins to foam, pour a cup of cold water into the pot. When it comes to the boil for the second time add another cup of water, repeating this process three times. Once the noodles are *al dente*, drain and rinse them immediately under cold water to prevent their sticking together. Make the miso broth, place the cold noodles in it and serve. You can cook more soba noodles than you will eat at one meal and store them in the fridge for later. This makes soba and miso broth an almost instant meal.

Thursday

Main meal   Fresh vegetables served either with tofu or chicken wok-fried in a little olive oil and served on a bed of steamed organic brown rice made from: 1 cup brown rice, 2–3 cups spring water, 2 tsp vegetable bouillon powder, 3 tbsp fresh parsley, 1 tsp marjoram, 2 cloves garlic. Wash the rice three times under running water and put into a saucepan. Boil the water in a kettle and pour over the rice. Add seasonings, except the parsley. Bring to the boil and cook gently for 45 minutes or until all the liquid has been absorbed. Garnish with parsley and serve. Follow with Apple Ginger Salad made from: 6 green apples, 1/4 cup fresh orange juice, 1 tsp grated fresh ginger, 2 tsp clear honey, 3 tbsp sesame seeds, toasted.

Light meal   Corn soup made from: 2 fresh corn on the cob, 300ml (1/2 pint) warm spring water, 2 spring onions, 1 tsp low-salt vegetable bouillon powder, 1/4 red pepper, 1/4 green pepper, a few sprigs of watercress, 1 tbsp tahini. Wash the corn and cut off the kernels. Add the water, spring onions and vegetable bouillon powder, season with tahini and blend until creamy in a blender or food processor. Sprinkle the peppers and watercress (chopped) on top. Serve with toast made from rye bread and spread with soya cottage cheese made from: 2 cups tofu, 3/4 cup mayonnaise, 1 tsp low-salt vegetable bouillon powder, 1 tsp caraway seeds, 1 tsp mild curry powder, 1 clove garlic, a handful of fresh herbs, 2 tbsp chopped chives. Mash the tofu well, add all the other ingredients and blend. This will keep for several days in the fridge.

Friday

Main meal   Dahl stew made from: $3/4$–1 cup red lentils or split peas, 1 large cauliflower, broken into florets, 3 large carrots, pinch of turmeric, 3 cloves garlic, 2 tbsp low-salt vegetable bouillon powder, 1 large onion, 1 red pepper, 1 yellow pepper, 2 tsp ground cumin, 2 tsp coriander, 2 tsp fresh ginger, 1–2 tsp mild curry powder, 1 large parsnip, 1 cup broccoli florets, 2 large tomatoes or 3 tbsp tomato paste with $1/2$ cup water. Put the lentils or peas into a large pot and cover with 3 cups water and 1 tablespoon low-salt vegetable bouillon powder. Cook for 45 minutes until tender. Purée in a food processor and set aside. While the peas are cooking, braise the onion in a little water with the garlic, turmeric, ginger and 1 tablespoon vegetable bouillon. When they have softened, add the vegetables, except the broccoli, and other seasonings and simmer until cooked. Pour the puréed legume mixture onto the vegetables, add the broccoli and serve immediately. Serve with a Sunshine Salad made from a few leaves of crisp lettuce, 1 medium sized fresh pineapple, 2 coarsely grated carrots, 2 finely chopped sticks celery, 2 handfuls sultanas, soaked, $1/2$ tsp celery seeds. Dress with Oil-free French Dressing made from: $3/4$ cup tomato juice, $1/4$ cup lemon juice or cider vinegar, 1 tsp whole-grain mustard, a little low-salt vegetable bouillon powder, 1 clove garlic, black pepper. Follow with Carob and Banana Ice-cream made from: 4 cups (about a litre) soya milk, 4 ripe bananas, 3 tbsp granular lecithin (optional), 1 cup unheated carob powder, $1/2$ cup pear concentrate, 1 tsp vanilla essence. Freeze the milk in a shallow plastic container. When frozen, remove from the freezer and leave for about half an hour until it is just soft enough to cut into slices. Put the bananas into the food processor, add about a cup of the frozen milk, the lecithin, carob powder, pear concentrate and vanilla, and blend until it is just mixed. Add the remainder of the soya milk. Should it become too liquid, return the mixture to the freezer for a few minutes, then stir before serving.

Light meal   Nut Milk Shake made from: $1/3$ cup almonds (blanched), $2/3$ cup soya milk, 5 pitted dates, a few drops vanilla essence, 1 tsp honey. Blend the almonds and the soya milk really well until the mixture is smooth. Add the other ingredients and process well. Serve immediately with an orange or apple.

Saturday

Main meal   Scrambled Tofu made from: $1/2$ cup diced onions, $1/2$ cup diced carrots, $1/2$ cup chopped celery, 2 cloves garlic, 1 tsp olive or soya oil, 2 cups mashed tofu, 1 tbsp soy sauce, 2 tsps low-salt vegetable bouillon powder, 1 teaspoon mild curry powder. Serve with Sprout Salad made from: 1 cup lentil sprouts, 1 cup fenugreek sprouts, 1 cup alfalfa sprouts, 1 cup shredded Chinese leaves, 3 sliced carrots, 4 diced tomatoes. Dress the salad with $1/2$ cup tofu or 3 medium-ripe tomatoes, $1/2$ cup fresh garden herbs, 1 tbsp sesame seeds, 2 tbsp lemon juice, 1 tsp onion powder, 1 tsp celery salt. Follow with fresh fruit salad with Cashew Cream made from: $1/2$ cup cashews, $3/4$ cup soya milk, dash of cinnamon or nutmeg. Put all ingredients in a food processor and blend well.

Light meal   Sprouted Lentil Salad made from: $1\tfrac{1}{2}$ cups fresh lentil sprouts, 1 large red pepper, 100 grams (4 oz) broccoli florets, 100 grams (4 oz) cauliflower florets, 175 grams (6 oz) button mushrooms, garnished with $1/4$ cup of splintered raw almonds and dressed with $1/4$ cup tomato juice, 2 tbsp cider vinegar, 1 tsp freshly grated root ginger, 2 tbsp fresh orange juice, 2 tsp vegetable bouillon powder or soy sauce, 1 tsp mild curry powder.

Sunday

Main meal   Spicy Shish-kebab made from: 1 large aubergine, chunks of tofu, 10 fresh tomatoes, 24 large mushrooms, 1 red pepper, 1 green pepper, 2 large onions, 1 large swede or 2 small turnips. Marinade: $1\tfrac{1}{4}$ cups olive oil, juice of 3 lemons, 2 tbsp red wine, 3 cloves garlic, 1 tsp coriander,

2 tbsp parsley, $1/2$ tsp nutmeg, 1 tbsp fresh basil, 1 tsp dried oregano. Place all the marinade ingredients together in a large bowl and mix thoroughly. Grill the aubergine until just soft and put with the rest of the vegetables into the marinade. Allow to sit for two to four hours. Skewer the vegetables and baste with the marinade as they are grilled. Serve with brown rice, or Kasha made from: 2 cups buckwheat, spring water to cover, 2 tsp vegetable bouillon powder, 2 tbsp chopped fresh parsley or other herbs. Place the buckwheat in a heavy-bottomed pan and roast it dry over a medium heat while stirring with a wooden spoon. As it begins to darken pour hot water over the buckwheat and add the vegetable bouillon powder and 1 tbsp of the herbs. Cover and simmer very slowly for about 15 to 20 minutes until all the liquid has been absorbed. Serve with remaining herbs as a garnish with a sliced tomato and fresh basil or parsley salad dressed with lemon, garlic and olive oil. Follow with Raspberry Ice-cream made from: 4 tbsp agar flakes, $2^1/2$ cups soya milk, $1/4$ cup apple-juice concentrate, 450 grams (1 lb) frozen raspberries. Place the agar flakes and soya milk in the top of a bain-marie and boil gently, stirring constantly until the agar is dissolved. Remove from the heat and pour in the apple-juice concentrate while still stirring. Add the raspberries, stir and chill. Stir the mixture from time to time until it has thickened, then freeze until firm.

Light meal Dairy-free muesli made from 2 tbsps oat flakes (or a combination of oat, rye and wheat) soaked overnight in a little spring water or fruit juice, a handful of raisins (also soaked overnight), grated apple or pear, juice of $1/2$ lemon, 3 tbsp soya milk or yoghurt, 1 tbsp apple concentrate or pear or strawberry juice, and $1/2$ tsp powdered cinnamon or ginger. Mix together the soaked oat flakes and raisins and combine with the grated apple or pear, lemon juice and the soya milk or yoghurt. Drizzle with fruit juice and sprinkle with fresh ground pecans, hazelnuts or three seeds (sesame, pumpkin and sunflower). Serve immediately.

Step Five
Go For Plant Power

PLANTS hold powerful medicine for women. It may seem unnecessary to state such an obvious truth, since every culture in the world from the beginning of human history has turned to herbs as medicine. Yet, as women in the post-industrial world, we find ourselves in the absurd position of having to rediscover our medicinal and health-promoting heritage not only by unearthing long-neglected local practices passed on verbally from woman to woman, but also by investigating herbal traditions from other parts of the world – Tibet, China, India, Japan and Native America. The benefits of making medicinal plants a part of your everyday life become clearer when you realise that the origins of most drugs lie in plants. Step Five explores how, when it comes to preventing or treating women's problems – from PMS to hot flushes – little works better or lasts longer than the gentle art of plant power.

Wise Woman Ways

Using plants and herbs for health and healing offers many advantages. First, their powers for enhancing health go far beyond their ability to alleviate symptoms. Wise women often use the whole of a plant, rejecting the preference of modern medicine for isolated active ingredients or drugs. In medicinal plants there are two kinds of compounds, each of which has an important part to play in treatment. The first are the active ingredients, the ones that capture the imagination of chemists and drug producers. The second are the compounds and substances which drug manufacturers ignore or eliminate but which wise women and good herbalists insist play a supportive role in healing. These compounds work synergistically with the active ingredients, making them easier for the body to use or dampening the action of what are often very potent plant chemicals, and thus helping to protect against side-effects. Some even prevent overdose by causing nausea if the body's safe level of tolerance is passed. It is the synergy of these primary active ingredients and their secondary helpers that makes herbs work so well.

There are many different substances and compounds in plants and herbs which have health-supporting abilities: the volatile oils, for instance, the tannins, alkaloids, bitters, glycosides and flavinoids. The most important for treating female problems and enhancing women's health are the *steroidal saponins*. The steroidal saponins fall into various categories. Some resemble cholesterol from which the body makes its own steroid hormones, the oestrogens, progesterone, and vitamin D. Others give the body a unique ability to regulate its own hormonal balance, probably because they provide the raw materials out of which the body can make whatever hormones it needs. These plants include many of the herbs long used by wise women to alleviate menstrual and menopausal problems, such as false unicorn root, black cohosh, blue cohosh, ginseng, fenugreek, squaw vine, liquorice and wild yam. Because of this balancing ability, unlike drugs or isolated ingredients, they are often used to treat two apparently opposite conditions. Ginseng, for example, can be used to treat both high and low blood pressure, and wild yam is a remedy for low progesterone as well as low oestrogen.

Preparations

Herbs can be taken in many different ways – as infusions, decoctions, syrups, tinctures, suppositories, capsules, and in baths, ointments and creams. You can grow your own herbs or buy them in bulk. Using the dried plant is by far the cheapest way to use herbs since you can buy a large amount at a time very cheaply and make up your own preparations. You can even buy empty gelatine capsules and fill them with a dried herb yourself. However, if you are a complete beginner it is probably easiest to rely on good-quality ready-made herbal products from a good supplier (see Resources) – whole herbs, herbs in capsules, herbal extracts and tinctures. Tinctures are made by using both water and alcohol to draw out and preserve a plant's chemical constituents. They are taken in a little water. They are best bought ready-made from a reputable supplier until you are more confident in the preparation of herbs, as each herb demands a specific ratio of water and alcohol to plant material. This ratio can be found in a pharmacopoeia. It is worth remembering that, just as people have different personalities, so do plants. Different plants sometimes work better for different people.

Infusions

These are made the way you would make a cup of tea, using the leaves, stems or flowers of a plant – whichever is appropriate. Take 25 grams (1 oz) of the dried herb or 50 grams (2 oz) of the fresh herb and put into a large teapot. Fill with boiling water, cover immediately and let it steep for ten to fifteen minutes. Or, to make one cup of infusion, take a teaspoon of the dried herb (two to three teaspoons of the fresh), pour a cup of boiling water over it, and allow to steep for ten to fifteen minutes. Strain and drink immediately or store for up to two days in a refrigerator and use as needed. Sometimes infusions are taken by the cupful, sometimes by the spoonful, depending upon the plant. A *decoction* is like a herbal infusion but is used to extract the goodness from the tougher parts of the plant, such as roots and barks. Rather than pouring boiling water over the herb and letting it steep, you put the herb in a pan with water and simmer it. Strain and drink as an infusion.

Tinctures

The part of the plant you are using can be fresh or dried, finely chopped or powdered. I prefer to use fresh plants in a ratio of 1:2 or one part of the plant to two parts of the fluid. If the plants are dried, the ratio becomes 1:5 as a general rule. In the case of camomile, for instance, use 200 grams (7 oz) of the dried flowers and pour over it 1 litre (1^3/4 pints) of the alcohol, the correct ratio of alcohol for this flower being forty-five per cent. The best alcohol for this purpose is vodka, but you can also use brandy, bearing in mind that sixty to seventy proof is equal to forty-five per cent alcohol. Put the mixture in an airtight container and allow it to macerate in a dark place away from direct sunlight for two to four weeks, shaking the jar thoroughly twice each day. Now the mixture is ready for pressing. Using a muslin bag or an old clean cloth, press as much of the fluid as you can from the herb, wasting as little as possible. You can use a cheese or a wine press to do this if you like. Then throw away the herb residue (it is great for making compost), pour the tincture into a dark bottle and store in a cool place. Tinctures will keep almost indefinitely, although I would never use one that is more than two years old.

Herbal Vinegars

Take a bottle of organic cider vinegar. Fill a jar with the part of the fresh plant you are using – root, rhizome, leaves, berries or flowers – cover with the vinegar and let it sit for six weeks. Vinegar must never be allowed to come in contact with metal, because it will corrode it, so cap the jar with plastic or protect the top with a piece of cellophane before closing. Vinegars can be taken by the spoonful mixed into a glass of spring water.

The Plants

Listed below is a small selection of herbs that are helpful for women. Get to know them; it is like making new friends. Each has its own personality and characteristics. All have been used for centuries to treat menstrual and menopausal complaints. The therapeutic actions of many have been scientifically validated.

Black Cohosh   *Cimicifuga racemosa*

Also known as squaw root, black snake root, or Sheng Ma in Chinese herbal medicine, this pungent root comes from the hardwood forests of North America. It has been used for hundreds of years by Native Americans to treat disorders of the womb, to promote and restore healthy menstruation, to soothe irritation and congestion in the cervix, womb and vagina, to relieve pains and to promote trouble-free delivery in childbirth – hence the name squaw root. It is one of the great plants for the management of menopause. Black cohosh contains phytoestrogens and has the ability to balance hormones in a woman's body. It can be particularly useful when a woman also suffers from aches and pains, anxiety, or stress. In one German study it was shown to relieve hot flushes, sleep disturbances and irritability as effectively as HRT but without dangerous side-effects.

How To Use   By decoction: one teaspoon of the dried root boiled in a cup of water for twelve minutes then allowed to cool and taken by the spoonful every few hours during the day. Tincture of the fresh root: ten to thirty drops in a little water sipped throughout the day.

What It Can Do
- Calm hot flushes and decrease their frequency. Rich in phyto-sterols and micronutrients, black cohosh helps the body to produce the hormones it needs to rebalance itself when used regularly over a few months.
- Ease aches and pains. The root contains compounds which help to relieve pain.
- Heighten energy and calm nerves. The root can raise the body's vital energies and improve the capacity to handle stress. Traditionally used to treat hysteria, it also reduces water retention.

- Help to prevent prolapses. The root has long been used in oriental medicine to correct prolapses of the womb and bladder.

Caution Black cohosh is never used to treat pregnant women or those suffering from menstrual flooding.

Sage *Salvia officianalis*

To Native Americans as well as the ancient Romans, sage was a sacred plant, burnt to cleanse both places and people. I use sage in its many forms all the time. For example, I often burn dried sage to cleanse the atmosphere of a room, calm stress, and heighten awareness. Its Latin name comes from *salvus*, meaning 'safe' or 'in good health'. Sage is a plant with an affinity for drying out that which is too wet. This is one of the reasons it can be so helpful in the treatment of night sweats and the kind of hot flushes that produce copious perspiration. Rich in phyto-sterols and flavonoids, it can be as effective as the synthetic oestrogens of HRT in banishing hot flushes. It is also used to treat infertility, is the best gargle for a sore throat you will find anywhere, and makes a great mouthwash. Sage is one of the easiest herbs to grow – it will thrive just about anywhere.

How To Use Make an infusion of one teaspoon of the dried leaves in a cup of water, let it sit for ten minutes then take one tablespoon of the cooled mixture one to eight times a day. Alternatively, use ten to twenty-five drops of tincture of sage every day. Also use sage in cooking, sprinkled on steamed or wok-fried vegetables and salads, in cooked grains, soups and casseroles.

What It Can Do

- Calm anxiety, banish depression and balance mood. A natural tranquilliser, rich in the calming minerals – magnesium, calcium and zinc, sage helps to calm the nerves and to create peaceful sleep. It can also balance emotions and banish emotional swings, largely because it helps to replenish minerals lost from the system.
- Reduce infection. Sage is one of the best herbs in the world

for enabling the body to overcome infections. Its essential oils concentrate in the urine, helping to clear infections there. Used as a mouthwash or a gargle, it can soothe a sore throat. Drunk as tea or taken as a tincture, it helps to banish infection in the body as a whole.

- Relieve headaches. Sage supports the liver and encourages good circulation, and many of the saponins it contains help to ease pain in the head.
- Banish night sweats and hot flushes. Often fast-acting, sage can relieve wet sweats day or night. Half a cup of sage tea taken at bedtime can work wonders for women who wake up drenched in sweat.
- Balance hormones in times of change. Sage has been used for thousands of years to help women going through major changes – easing their first period, increasing fertility, making menopause a smooth transition – thanks to its ability to balance hormones.
- Improve digestion and strengthen the liver. The volatile essential oil of sage contains chemicals which help both the stomach and the liver to produce more enzymes, thus improving digestion and preventing nausea and wind.
- Relieve flooding and menstrual cramps. Sage's tannins and volatile oil relieve pain in the womb and help to dry up excessive flow.
- Rejuvenate the body. A natural anti-ager, sage is full of anti-oxidants, antiseptics and minerals. It has been used for generations to protect hair from greying and skin from wrinkling, not to mention helping to prevent cancer and other degenerative conditions.
- Ease inflammation and clear joint pains. Its phyto-hormones help to oil the joints and dissolve mineral deposits there and to relieve aches and pains.

Caution   Sage is a drying herb and as such should not be used by a woman who is experiencing vaginal dryness or a dry mouth. It is a herb to use frequently when needed but not continuously over long periods of time or it may lose its effectiveness.

Motherwort *Leonurus cardiaca*

Also called lion's tail or Yi Mu Cao in the Chinese Pharmacopoeia, motherwort grows in waste places. Traditionally used
for reducing anxiety during pregnancy, the plant has good
sedative properties which have been well validated by scientific
experiments. It calms the nervous system while acting as a
tonic to the whole body. Its leaves are full of mind-altering
natural chemicals which studies in China have shown to have
a regulating effect on the womb and the heart, bringing calm
in its wake. This is one of the reasons why, in addition to being
used by women to ease hot flushes, banish insomnia, and
restore elasticity to the walls of the vagina, it is an excellent
herb for the treatment of many heart conditions. It is the most
physically and psychologically comforting plant I know.

How To Use Motherwort is rich in alkaloids and is bitter
when drunk as an infusion. It is easier to take as a tincture
or as a herbal vinegar. Take ten to twenty-five drops of the
tincture made from the fresh plant every two to six hours or
one to two teaspoons of the herb vinegar as desired.

What It Can Do
- Calm the nerves. There is something very calming and
  balancing about motherwort that is hard to describe to those
  who have never used it. Taken frequently it can relieve
  anxiety, nourish the nervous system and relax tensions, and
  at the same time act as an energy-boosting tonic. It is an
  excellent herb to take just before and during times of stress.
- Minimise hot flushes. The herb can reduce the intensity,
  length and frequency of hot flushes, even helping to calm
  the dizziness or faintness that can accompany them. For
  best results it should be used regularly for twelve weeks
  or longer, but sometimes ten drops or so of the tincture
  in a little spring water can ease a hot flush while it is
  happening.
- Promote undisturbed sleep. This herb is a wonderful help
  when you wake in the night with sweats and have trouble

dropping off again. Keep the tincture beside the bed with a glass of spring water and take ten to twenty drops of the tincture each time you wake up. It will even help to banish anxiety and bad dreams.

● Eliminate water retention. A little motherwort taken every few hours acts as a natural diuretic.

● Tone up womb and vagina. By improving circulation and thickening tissues which have lost their elasticity and tone, the herb can rejuvenate the tissues of the bladder, womb and vagina when taken a couple of times a day for two to four weeks.

● Relieve cramps. The best remedy for menstrual cramps when the menstrual flow is light to moderate or even absent. Take five to ten drops of the tincture or half to one teaspoon of the vinegar every few minutes until the cramps have gone and repeat as necessary. Prolonged use strengthens the muscles of the womb and makes it resistant to cramping in the future.

Caution Motherwort should not be used when a woman is experiencing menstrual flooding since it can aggravate this tendency.

Ginseng *Panax ginseng*

Oriental ginseng, widely cultivated in China, Korea, Japan and Russia, is probably the most studied plant in modern times. More potent and effective than its American cousin *panax quinquefolium*, it has been praised for centuries for its rejuvenating properties, its ability to protect against illness, to enhance the body's ability to handle stress – even to prolong life. The herb is a great ally, the most effective herb for treating very severe symptoms in menopausal women. Many of ginseng's benefits will be lost if you take more than 2 grams a day of vitamin C; taking vitamin E will enhance its action. The most effective ginseng is the dried root, which you chew, or a good tincture made from it. Ginseng should be chosen carefully, as there are a lot of relatively worthless types on the market. Research has shown that for ginseng to work it has to be replete with *ginsenosides*, the active compounds from the plant. Ginseng can heighten immunity, improve the functions of the heart and lungs, counter fatigue and balance female hormones through its oestrogenic action.

How To Use   Always buy the best ginseng you can afford and take it either as a fresh root tincture (five to twenty drops one to three times a day), as an infusion or tea (25 grams [1 oz] of the dried root in a cup of water a day), or by chewing on a piece of the root the size of the tip of your little finger every day. The effects of ginseng are cumulative, so you need to take it for six to eight weeks in order to feel its full benefits.

What It Can Do

- Regulate hormones and banish menstrual flooding. Rich in phyto-sterols, ginseng encourages the body to produce the oestrogen and progesterone it needs, along with other steroid hormones, gradually enabling the hormone system to completely rebalance itself. This can be particularly helpful in the years just before menopause; it can balance menstrual flow and prevent flooding up to menopause.

- Enhance the capacity to handle stress. Nothing can compare with ginseng's adaptogenic abilities to strengthen the adrenals, protect from exhaustion, and support the function of glands such as the thyroid, pituitary and hypo-thalamus involved in stress protection. Ginseng banishes fatigue and slowly rebuilds stamina and energy.

Echinacea   *Echinacea purpurea*

Purple cone flower or Black Sampson is a plant native to the prairies of North America with unequalled properties to stim-ulate the immune system, heal wounds, enhance skin, counter infection and calm inflammation. The Sioux used it for snake bites, blood poisoning and wound healing. Until the twentieth century its roots and rhizomes were used for the treatment of fever and infections from flu and colds to serious conditions such as typhoid, meningitis, malaria, diphtheria, boils and abscesses. With the advent of large-scale drug manufacturing, the beautiful echinacea plant was almost forgotten – except in Germany. There, researchers began to quantify its effects on the body, discovering that it has properties equal to and often greater than most antibiotics to prevent and heal infection. Echinacea is a plant product I would never want to be without. I use it to protect from infection through the long dark winters and to treat illness in myself and my family.

How To Use The ground herb can be taken in capsule form – one to four capsules three to four times a day – depending on whether it is being used for protection or to treat illness. Take fifteen to fifty drops of the fresh plant tincture in a little water once or twice a day for prevention, or several times a day as treatment – up to two teaspoons an hour for a day or two at the onset of illness.

What It Can Do
- Insure against illness and premature ageing. Used throughout periods of stress, echinacea reinforces the body's defence mechanisms and heightens immunity, warding off colds and flu and other minor illnesses.
- Boost immunity when illness strikes. The immunity-enhancing qualities of echinacea make it a potent ally in fighting off viral or bacterial infections, including boils, abscesses and carbuncles, as well as healing wounds.
- Protect skin and body from degeneration. Hyaluronic acid forms a barrier against infection and helps to keep skin strong, resilient and youthful. As the body ages, an enzyme attacks the hyaluronic acid, and it changes from a firm jelly into a thin watery fluid. Echinacea prevents the enzyme from attacking, thus inhibiting the spread of infection and maintaining firm skin.

Caution   Like many plants, echinacea should not be used continuously, because the body can become accustomed to it and this may negate some of its potent health-enhancing properties.

Goldenseal *Hydrastis canadensis*

Favourite cure-all of the Cherokee Indians, goldenseal has in recent years won praise from scientists for its widespread benefits, which include relieving nausea, calming digestive disturbances, and banishing skin diseases and haemorrhoids. It can be used as a douche in the treatment of vaginal infections, as a mouthwash in the treatment of gum problems and to fight off flu and fevers. One of the most generally effective of all remedies, this is another herb I would never want to be without.

How To Use Use the powdered root, preferably in capsules rather than as an infusion, since goldenseal has an unpleasant taste. Take one to four capsules three times a day, or ten to thirty drops of the fresh herb tincture three or four times a day.

What It Can Do

- Soothe digestion and relieve liver problems. A bitter tonic, goldenseal was much used in the nineteenth century to ease disorders of the stomach and heal the liver. The alkaloids which the root contains not only stimulate bile production and secretion but destroy unhelpful bacteria in the gut and increase the tone and movement of the gastrointestinal tract. The root relieves nausea during pregnancy, has overall tonic actions on the nervous system and, applied in strong infusion, is an excellent treatment for eczema and many other skin problems.
- Counter infection. Effective against all kinds of infection, goldenseal can banish catarrh in the head and throat, and clear up infections of the teeth and gums when used as a mouthwash.
- Calm uterine contractions. Gently strengthening muscle tone and circulation, goldenseal has a mildly sedative and muscle-relaxing effect on the body and helps to stabilise blood sugar. It can be used for menstrual disorders, especially menorrhagia.

Caution This should not be taken during pregnancy.

Chastetree *Vitex agnus castus*

Also called monk's pepper, this plant was named for its ability to calm the lascivious desires of men. For most women, however, it has the exact opposite effect, stimulating libido and energising the whole system while balancing emotions. Chastetree is more helpful and far-reaching in its effects than any other plant for peri-menopausal, menopausal and post-menopausal women. It works superbly, whether hormones are deficient or in excess, by acting on the pituitary to harmonise imbalances. What is wonderful about the berries is that it is hard take them in excess; the herb never forces the body to make more of any particular hormone than it needs. Chastetree is far better known in Europe and the Far East than in Britain and the Americas. Its berries have been used for centuries to protect from and even to help to cure cancers of the breasts and womb, to reduce breast lumps and tenderness, countcract oedema, clear skin problems, moisten dry vaginal tissues and banish hot flushes, as well as eliminating menstrual cramps and restoring emotional calm. Chastetree is not rich in phyto-hormones, relying on its glycosides, micronutrients and flavonoids to work its wonders, so be patient. It has profound effects on the body and psyche, but this takes time. An improvement can be expected after eight or twelve weeks of daily use. After about a year to eighteen months you will probably find that you no longer need to use the plant.

How To Use As an infusion: drink one cup of tea a day made from the freshly ground berries. In powdered form, in capsules: one capsule three to four times a day. You can also take fifteen drops to one teaspoon of the tincture one to three times a day.

What It Can Do
- Eliminate hot flushes. Research carried out in Germany has shown that the berry can stimulate progesterone synthesis and secretion and balance the excess oestrogen which can cause flushes in some women.

- Regulate periods and banish cramping, endometriosis and fibroids. Whether the problem is spotting, flooding, or irregular periods, this plant can help thanks to its action on the pituitary. Chastetree's anti-inflammatory properties can also help to shrink fibroids when the plant is used regularly for twelve to thirty-six months.
- Keep the vagina moist. Through its oestrogen-balancing abilities, chastetree helps to regulate vaginal secretions while offering protection from oestrogen-dominant illnesses such as cancer.
- Strengthen bones. Its capacity to increase progesterone production makes this herb an important ally against osteoporosis and it may even help to reverse bone-loss.
- Ease constipation and digestive problems. Sluggish digestion is no match for the chasteberry, which helps to restore digestion easily and permanently provided you take it for long enough. It can also clear up skin problems that develop as a result of hormonal change, and can banish fluid retention with regular use.
- Eliminate depression and balance mood. Typical PMS symptoms, ranging from migraines and depression to ordinary headaches and anxiety, can yield slowly but permanently to chastetree. This usually takes about six months and it is wise to continue the treatment for a further six months at least to make benefits permanent.

Dong Quai *Angelica sinensis*

This is the most prized of all the oriental plant treatments for women's hormonal problems, acting as a sister to ginseng. Although its oestrogen content is a mere 0.25 per cent of that of oestrogen-based drugs, studies have shown that this root can quickly stop hot flushes which result from too little or the wrong kinds of oestrogen in the body, and perform many other useful tasks: it can reduce high blood pressure, fight bacteria and viruses, counteract water retention, calm menopausal anxiety, stimulate a sluggish metabolism, protect the cardiovascular system, and eliminate insomnia, nervousness and depression. This remedy works fast – usually in a week or two. It is often more effective when used in conjunction with ginseng, since they perfectly balance each other. Western herbal practitioners some-imes suggest taking Dong Quai for a fortnight then ginseng for the next fortnight to reap the highest benefits from both.

How To Use   As with ginseng, a thin slice of dried root can be chewed three times a day. As an infusion, take half to one cup a day. Fifteen to thirty drops of the fresh root tincture can be taken one to three times a day.

What It Can Do
- Improve sleep. Rich in calming minerals like magnesium and in phyto-hormones, Dong Quai can be very effective against the sleeplessness in menopause. It calms nerves and alleviates mood swings in the daytime too.
- Moisten the vagina. Known for its ability to ease vaginal dryness, Dong Quai soothes the whole of the pelvis, relieving cramps and aches and restoring warmth and vitality to the tissues.
- Ease hot flushes. Fast-working, this root is excellent for treating hot flushes, particularly in those who are chilly by nature. It is not the plant of choice for women who tend to be very warm, however, since taking it can make you warmer.
- Rejuvenate skin. This plant enhances the flow of blood to the skin and brings a glow to the face, smoothing out fine lines and thickening skin that has thinned from age. It also thickens the walls of the vagina and bladder and relieves many rheumatic aches and pains.

Caution   Dong Quai is not a remedy to use if you regularly have bloating, menstrual flooding or diarrhoea, or if you have fibroids. Neither should it be used if you are using blood-thinning herbs or aspirin. Its use should be discontinued if there is any tenderness or discomfort in the breasts.

Wild Yam *Dioscorea villosa*

There are many related species of the *dioscoriaceae* family which have similar properties to *villosa*, including *Discorea mexicana*. Wild yam was traditionally used to prevent miscarriage, as a natural tonic, and for natural birth control without side-effects, as it does not interfere with normal periods. The whole plant, which supplies the raw materials for the body to make hormones, has much to offer perimenopausal, menopausal and post-menopausal women. It soothes the nerves, eases menstrual pains and encourages the production of progesterone, countering oestrogen-dominance and the many conditions associated with it. It is effective against intestinal wind, colic and nausea, and it stimulates the libido in many women. The root has also been shown to lower blood cholesterol and high blood pressure.

How To Use Take an infusion of the dried root – half to one cup once or twice a day – or a tincture of the dried root – ten to thirty drops three or four times a day. You can also take the ground root in capsules. Wild yam cream, which contains converted natural progesterone, can be used on the body; it acts as an antidote to osteoporosis and can reverse bone loss after it has occurred (see Step Eight).

What It Can Do
- Ease joint and muscle pains and headaches. The root is one of the best anti-inflammatory plants known to man.
- Reverse osteoporosis. Wild yam cream is full of naturally derived progesterone which increases the rate of bone formation. As John Lee writes in *The Lancet* of 24 November 1990: 'the signs and symptoms of osteoporosis cleared in every patient [using the wild yam cream] and the incidence of fractures dropped to zero.'
- Moisten the vagina. Thanks to its hormone-balancing capacities, taken internally, wild yam helps to calm itching and burning in the genitals of menopausal and post-menopausal women. Wild yam cream with natural proges-

terone is also effective in this respect if applied directly to the vagina and the genital area.

● Banish PMS and menstrual pain. Its ability to stimulate the production of progesterone in a woman's body makes wild yam enormously helpful in soothing the nerves, easing menstrual pain, preventing flooding, and countering PMS in most women.

Age of Treason

Orthodox medicine's almost total disregard for the use of phyto-hormone-rich plants in the treatment of women's ailments is of recent origin. It is as though with the coming of patentable drugs, centuries of traditional methods were dismissed with the wave of a hand. 'Uterine tonics' made from hormone-rich herbs and plants were used for centuries to treat all manner of female complaints. They still work. Once you get to know the actions of various herbs – and the best way of doing this is to use them or to observe their effect on other people – you begin to develop a feel for the character of each herb and a skill that enables you to call on the plant or plants you need just when you need them. But it is important to remember that plants are slower-acting than drugs, so you need to be patient. It is often necessary to use a herb for a few weeks or even longer before you will experience its full benefits. However, I have frequently found that a herb will bring almost immediate relief. One big advantage of using herbs is that many, when taken over a period of time, will do their job so well that you will not have to use them again. Another important thing to remember when using herbs is that they often work well in combination.

It is essential that the supply of herbs you are using is clean, preferably organically grown. Some herbs on the market today have been grown in countries where pesticides and herbicides are sprayed heavily. Others are either not fresh or have been irradiated or contaminated with chemicals. Often even the suppliers themselves are not aware how the dried plants have been handled. Once you have your herbs it is a good idea to keep them in air-tight jars in the refrigerator, so they stay potent for as long as possible.

Having worked and played with plants, herbs and tinctures for many years, I have developed the deepest respect for their beauty and their power. Each plant has its own unique personality which you can turn to for health or strength when you need it. I grow herbs in my garden, and use them fresh in summer and dried in winter for everything from cooking soups and making salads to healing coughs, banishing headaches and cleansing the atmosphere of a room. I also keep a whole row of litre and half-litre bottles of plant tinctures just behind my desk in the room in which I work and call on them frequently when help is needed – for energy, to calm stress or to ward off an impending infection. The bottom line is this: the support which plants can give a woman on her natural menopause journey is nothing short of miraculous.

Step Six
Banish Bad Blood

MOUNTING xenoestrogenic pollution in our environment and the widespread use of artificial hormones for birth control and HRT have produced an epidemic of female problems arising from oestrogen-dominance in the body. The stage has been set for the development of a 'bad blood' plague. It is a plague which only women themselves will be able to defeat, first by becoming aware of its causes and then by taking action against it, personally and politically. Step Six examines some of the most common bad blood conditions now appearing in ever greater numbers, the treatments offered, and ways women can counter these problems for themselves.

Endometriosis

A mysterious and rapidly increasing condition of modern times in the Western world, endometriosis is where, instead of breaking down and being shed fully during a menstrual period, the normal endometrium or uterine lining which develops each month proliferates inside the uterine cavity. Tiny islets of endometrial tissue can migrate to other areas of the pelvis, the fallopian tubes, the surface of the ovaries – and occasionally beyond – to the sides of the pelvic wall and occasionally onto the bowel. Because they are of the same endometrial tissue as that in the womb, they swell and diminish with the ebb and flow of monthly hormones, then are painfully shed at the time of the period. Endometriosis can be accompanied by pelvic pain, cramps, infertility and disturbed menstrual cycles. Pain is often worse at ovulation and just before and during a period. The only sure way to diagnose the condition is via *laparoscopy* although sometimes endometrial lesions can be seen during a pelvic examination of the vagina, vulva or cervix. Often endometriosis and fibroids are found together. The incidence of endometriosis has increased dramatically in recent years, partly because women are giving birth later and having fewer children, and because of widespread oestrogen dominance. For oestrogen is the hormone of proliferation, responsible for the build-up of endometrial tissue. When it gets out of hand endometriosis can be one of the results.

Common Treatment

The standard medical treatments for endometriosis include taking birth control pills, using a progestogen to suppress menstruation, prescribing analgesics and narcotics to kill the pain, or drugs which in effect render a woman menopausal so long as she takes them. Other drugs commonly used for the treatment of endometriosis can bring masculinisation, such as facial hair growth. None of these treatments have been shown to be very successful. Surgery is another standard treatment for endometriosis, either to remove the endometrial lesions themselves or, more radically, a complete hysterectomy and ovary removal. The cause of endometriosis is much debated. Since adequate progesterone inhibits the proliferation of endometrial tissue, it is not surprising that a growing number of doctors, nutritionists and naturopaths prefer to recommend the cyclic use of natural progesterone so that the pain and menstrual flow are adequately reduced and the need for surgery eliminated.

Look Within

Endometriosis is often called 'the career woman's ailment', because there is often a conflict between the sufferer's unfulfilled desires and what she has chosen to do or feels obliged to do in terms of her day-to-day life. A woman's inner self can use this condition to demand attention, through pain or abnormal menstrual cycles, asking her to turn back from total absorption in the externals of her life and look within.

When endometriosis makes life miserable, take a little time for yourself and write down exactly how you are feeling – both physically and emotionally. This works best if it is done without paying much attention to what you are writing or trying to make sense of anything – just letting the words pour out of you. You may be surprised by some of the impulses and desires that are expressed. See what can be done gradually to create space for yourself. Do you need more time alone? Do you need to allow yourself more freedom of self-expression in your work? Your relationships? Are you in need of self-care? Time off? Are you resting enough? What changes would you like to see in your life if anything were possible? Are you living somebody else's values – your parents', your boss', your family's – rather than your own? Do you feel helpless, a victim of your condition and your pain, or do you accept the possibility that you can change your life?

Castor-oil Packs

Castor-oil packs are an age-old remedy traditionally used to treat everything from colitis and peptic ulcers to arthritis, and female problems from back pains to fibroids, PMS and endometriosis. They work. Preliminary research at the George Washington School of Medicine in the United States has shown that they are likely to improve the functioning of the immune system. They are an excellent treatment for endometriosis, not only to alleviate discomfort but to speed recovery. Use them at least three times a week – preferably every day.

You will need:

- cotton or wool flannel cloth (a piece of old sheet is fine but make sure there are no synthetics in the fabric)
- plastic freezer bag or plastic sheet
- hot water bottle

- two safety pins
- 150 grams (6oz) of castor oil
- a bath towel
- baking soda

Your cloth needs to be big enough so that, folded twice (i.e. with four thicknesses of cloth), it is about 25 centimetres (10 inches) wide and 30 centimetres (12 inches) long. Fold your cloth and pour castor oil over it so that it is saturated with the oil but not dripping. While lying down, apply it to the abdomen, then lay the plastic bag or sheet over the soaked cloth. Put the hot water bottle on top – it should be as warm as possible – then cover with the towel folded lengthways over the whole area. Leave the castor-oil pack on for a minimum of an hour – all night if you can manage it. Afterwards cleanse the skin using water to which a teaspoon of baking soda has been added. Provided it is kept clean, the soaked flannel can be used many times.

Herb Help

Two herbs are traditionally used with success in the treatment of endometriosis: raspberry leaves and chastetree or *Vitex agnus-castus*. They work well together.

- Raspberry leaf tea is easy to make. Simply steep a tablespoon of the dried herb in a pint of hot water for five minutes and drink hot or cold throughout the day with a little honey if you like.
- *Vitex agnus-castus* can be taken in the form of fresh powdered berries (three capsules a day with food), as tea made from the powdered berries or – easiest of all – in tincture form: twenty drops in a little water two to three times a day.

Chastetree is slow-acting but profound in its effects. It has a reputation for being virtually free of side-effects. It is an enormously useful natural remedy for severe hot flushes, and can help to eliminate flooding, spotting, irregular cycles, fibroids and endometriosis while balancing emotions, making skin clearer and improving vaginal dryness. It also counters most of the usual PMS problems, from headaches and depression to water retention and breast tenderness. I first learned the virtues of *agnus castus* from Dr Dagmar Liechti von Brasch. Dr Liechti was the niece of the famous natural Swiss physician Max Bircher Benner, who founded the Bircher Benner Clinic in Zurich. Dr Liechti was head of the clinic for forty years, during which time she gave birth to and raised five children and ran a big hospital. Chastetree was her preferred remedy for menopausal women because it was so successful on so many levels. A conventionally trained medical doctor, she had at her disposal every possible natural and hormonal treatment, yet she most often opted for this one. Results begin to show in two or three months of daily use and can become permanent after a year.

Diet

Throw out all your coffee, sugar, colas, dairy products – cut out all milk and milk products – and anything containing hydrogenated oils, such as margarines, junk fats, cooking oils and convenience foods. Eliminate shellfish. Eat fifty per cent of your foods raw, especially fruits and vegetables, and make sure you eat plenty of high-fibre whole grains, lentils and beans. Avoid red meat, but use organic tofu often as a protein food. Have a green drink – chlorella, spirulina, green barley or wheatgrass in water – or fresh vegetable juice daily.

Progesterone

Take progesterone either as a cream rubbed on the skin twice a day, or in oil form, taken under the tongue, from day ten or twelve to day twenty-six of your menstrual cycle. John Lee says, 'I recommend that a woman increase the dose of the cream until she is satisfied her pelvic pains are decreasing. Once that dose is reached, a woman can continue for three to five years before gradually lowering it.' Lee finds that this decreases menstrual flow and gives the body time to heal the endometrial lesions. If the pains come back he advises women to continue the treatment until menopause. Lee has treated patients with mild to moderate endometriosis in this manner for the past thirteen years and none of them has ever had to resort to surgery. Alternate the sites at which you apply the cream – breasts, back, belly, face, neck, thighs – and use at least one 50-gram (2-oz) jar each month between days ten and twenty-six of your cycle. Progesterone oil can be useful when symptoms are severe, since it contains high levels of progesterone. Put four or five drops of the oil under the tongue and keep it in the mouth for at least five minutes without swallowing (this takes a bit of practice). Increase or decrease the dosage of the oil or cream depending upon the severity of the symptoms and on how rapidly the cream is absorbed.

Fibroid Tumours

Fibroids are benign (non-cancerous) tumours of the uterus. Made out of lumps of fibrous tissue very much like the tissue of the womb itself, they grow into unusual shapes which either lace the lining of the womb or are attached by a stump to its outer walls. Fifty per cent of women in the West are thought to have fibroids although most women are unaware of having them. They are more common in black women than in white and they usually develop in the eight to ten years before menopause. The size of fibroids can vary from tiny to massive. A single fibroid can weigh as much as a newborn baby. (The largest ever recorded in medical history weighed 36 kilos (80 lb)!

Only if fibroids cause trouble will a doctor consider removing them, as a rule. Many women with fibroids have no symptoms at all. Others experience menstrual cramps, pelvic pains, pressure on the bladder or rectum, a swollen belly, or extremely heavy periods which can result in long-term fatigue and anaemia. When a woman's hormones are fluctuating wildly, as they can do in the years just before menopause or when she is under a lot of stress, fibroids can grow quickly, sometimes even causing haemorrhaging. Fibroids are responsible for a third of women's gynaecological problems and are the most common reason that hysterectomies are performed, because they can be hard to remove without taking out the womb. Occasionally fibroids are removed without taking out the uterus through an operation called a *myomectomy*, but this is generally done only when there is a single large fibroid present or when a woman wants to become pregnant, since the operation is difficult. Fibroids are very rarely cancerous.

Fibroids have a tendency to grow and shrink as a woman's hormone levels shift during her monthly cycles. Highly oestrogen-dependent, they are most prevalent in oestrogen-dominant women, particularly women who have not had children early on in life and are in their late thirties or forties. The good news is that once menopause arrives and oestrogen levels drop sharply, fibroids become so small that often they can no longer be detected by pelvic examination. The presence of fibroids in a woman is usually confirmed by a *sonogram* or *ultrasound* since it can be difficult for a doctor to distinguish between an ovarian growth and a fibroid through pelvic examination alone.

Common Treatment

Until recently the best treatment for most fibroids – unless causing excessive discomfort – has been to watch and wait for them to disappear with the onset of menopause, provided of course that the woman has not been given oestrogen replacement. Now doctors at the forefront of the natural menopause revolution urge women to make dietary changes and recommend the use of progesterone cream or oil. A few prescribe oral doses of progesterone.

Look Within

In some women fibroids almost seem a physical manifestation of plans, projects or dreams that have either outlived their usefulness or have not yet been fulfilled. Fibroids can be like frustrated creative energy stuck in the womb. It can be useful to take a look at your life and ask yourself if a job, a project or a relationship has outlived its value. Have you in some way outgrown the life you are living? If so, would you like to change things? Sometimes fibroids are linked with conflicts over whether or not to have a child, or intimate relationships.

Castor-oil Packs

Use three times a week or more when there is any discomfort, heavy bleeding, abdominal pressure or other symptoms (see above).

Epsom Salts Baths

Take long Epsom salts baths regularly. Pour two cups of household grade Epsom salts (available from the chemist) into the bath and fill it with blood-heat water. Then immerse yourself for twenty to thirty minutes, topping up with warm water when necessary to maintain a comfortable temperature. Afterwards, lie down for fifteen minutes. Better still, have an Epsom salts bath just before you go to bed.

Herb Help

Lady's mantle (*Alchemilla vulgaris*) tincture is an old natural treatment for fibroids traditionally used by herbalists. Chastetree (*Vitex agnus-castus*) is also useful, as is a combination of mistletoe and butterbur.

- Lady's mantle (*Alchemilla vulgaris*) is said to have magical properties offering support to women either entering or leaving the role of motherhood. It is also good for excessive menstrual flow and flooding taken as a tea (25 grams [1 oz] of the dried herb to one pint of boiling water) or in tincture form (ten to twenty-five drops several times a day). Lady's mantle is excellent for relieving headaches, too.
- Chastetree (*Vitex agnus-castus*) berries (see above) are effective in tincture form (ten to twenty drops two to three times a day). Both chastetree and lady's mantle are anti-oestrogenic in their actions. They can be profitably used together.

- A combination of mistletoe (*Viscus album*) and butterbur (*Petasites hybrids*) is one of the best herbal remedies for shrinking fibroids. Developed by the Swiss physician Dr Alfred Vogel, it is available in most countries in the form of *Petasan Tincture*, made by Bioforce. Normal dosage is ten to twenty drops three times a day.

Caution The Chinese herb Dong Quai (*Angelica sinensis*) which in general is excellent for many female problems, should not be used if you have fibroids, since it has been shown to increase their size in some women. Avoid oestrogen replacement too, as this also increases their growth.

Diet

Whole grains are full of lignins, compounds which have an anti-oestrogenic effect on the body. Eat plenty of rye, millet, soya products, oats, buckwheat, barley, corn and brown rice. Sprinkle two tablespoons of fresh flaxseeds ground in a coffee grinder over porridge in the morning or over a salad. Reduce your fat intake to fifteen to twenty per cent of your calories. Try to take fifty per cent of your foods raw. Avoid coffee, cocoa, chocolate or sugar and keep away from junk fats – from margarines to golden cooking oils – and from anything which contains trans fatty acids: no junk foods or fried foods.

Progesterone

Provided dietary changes are also made, when enough prog-esterone is supplied, fibroid growth is arrested and frequently reversed as well. Good herbal support (see above) works well with both. Progesterone cream should be rubbed on different areas of the skin twice a day. It can also be used in oil form taken under the tongue from day twelve to day twenty-six of your menstrual cycle. You should use up a 50-gram (2-oz) jar during this two-week period. Vary the sites at which you apply the cream: breasts, back, belly, face, neck and thighs. It is always worthwhile for your doctor to monitor the results of such natural treatment by way of regular sonogram tests three or four times a year to verify shrinkage. Progesterone plays an important emotional role in women with fibroids by helping to soften the frustration or anger often associated with them. This is thanks to progesterone's role as a precursor to important brain chemicals and stress hormones.

Vaginal Irritation, Dryness and Thinning

At menopause some women experience a thinning of the vaginal walls, which can lead to irritation and in a few cases even to repeated urinary infection. This thinning of the walls of the vagina and the symptoms that can accompany it – referred to by the patriarchal medical experts as *atrophic vaginitis* or *vulval dystrophy* – are by no means inevitable. Many women, especially those who are physically active and have active sex lives, never experience it at all. Others have had a tendency to dryness since their twenties, whatever their lifestyle.

Look Within

Do not allow yourself to feel that you are some kind of freak or growing old, or incapable of enjoying intercourse. Many women never give full vent to the power of their sexuality nor experience the full flood of the pleasure an abandoned sexual encounter can bring until menopause, when they are free of fear of pregnancy. Vaginal thinning, which is a natural part of lowered oestrogen levels in menopausal women, can easily be treated without resorting to potentially dangerous hormone drugs. So if you have been feeling timid or negative about yourself, set those feelings aside and do something about it.

Herb Help

Stay away from soaps, bubble baths, shower gels, and nylon tights or underwear: all of these things can make this condition worse. There are several herbs which treat it very effectively: motherwort and chastetree (taken internally), along with calendula, aloe vera and comfrey (used externally). They can also help to prevent recurrent vaginal and bladder infections.

- Taking a tincture of motherwort (fifteen to twenty drops in a glass of water several times a day) is an excellent way of restoring thickness to vaginal tissues and remoisturising the vagina.

- While chastetree was used in the Middle Ages to calm the lascivious thoughts of celibate monks (hence its name), it has a powerful stimulating effect on women's libido when taken over a few months. It is also excellent for improving moisture and circulation in vaginal tissues. Take the berries in tincture form (ten to twenty drops two or three times a day).

- Calendula (*Calendula officinalis*) in a good cream base (see Resources) can help to soften and toughen the tissues of the vagina and the vulva. It can also relieve itching if applied three times a day, and protect against infection.

- In a cream base (see Resources) comfrey (*Symphytum officinale*) is the best soother of all for itchy vaginal tissue. It can also be used as a lubricant instead of the usual Vaseline or KY Jelly during intercourse. Use it three times a day for three months and you may never need to use it again.

- Pure aloe vera juice is useful when vaginal tissues have become hot, dry and uncomfortable. Simply wipe it on several times a day.

Premenstrual Syndrome

PMS is a major problem. Today somewhere between forty and sixty per cent of menstruating women in the Western world suffer to some degree from premenstrual syndrome. There are no specific laboratory tests for PMS. Neither are there specific clinical signs for the condition, which is why it is called a syndrome – a set of complex symptoms which occur together and don't appear to have one specific cause. Women with PMS can experience symptoms from bloating and depression to mood swings, headaches, weight gain, irritability, fatigue and lack of interest in sex. The symptoms usually begin a week or more before a period starts and last for two or three days into the period before they clear.

Look Within

The causes of PMS are many: some are nutritional, others psychological, many are stress-related. Even a woman's attitude towards menstruation plays a part in PMS. In our culture menstruation has long been associated with the work of the devil. It is often called 'the curse'. The whole female cycle involving the build-up and flow of blood has been regarded with disgust. Women often feel humiliated or grow up fearing there is something diseased and unclean about their body. Exercise is important in the treatment of PMS, not only because of the physical benefits that regular exercise brings, but also because it can enhance self-esteem and erase the old pattern of feeling like a victim going through monthly suffering.

Herb Help

There are a number of herbs which bring potent help to a woman wrestling with PMS. Some of the best are motherwort, wild yam (either *Dioscorea villosa* or *Dioscorea mexicana*), black cohosh and Dong Quai.

- Motherwort (*Leonurus cardiaca*) is my favourite plant for PMS, particularly for the emotional ups and downs. Ten to twenty drops of tincture of motherwort works wonders when you are feeling unsettled. Alternatively, you can take five to fifteen drops of the tincture every day for a month or two to stabilise emotions in the long term. Motherwort is the most comforting herb I have ever come across. It brings a sense of inner security and calm strength that is unequalled by anything except perhaps a love affair – maybe not even that.
- Wild yam (*Dioscorea villosa* or *Dioscorea mexicana*), from which so many hormones are derived, is the most effective single herb for treating PMS in most women. Taking three grams of powdered wild yam a day, split into two doses,

and making improvements to diet and lifestyle often works so well that, unless a woman is seriously oestrogen-dominant, PMS can be banished permanently. And the nice thing about using wild yam is that after taking it for three to six months, many women find they can stop using it altogether without a return of symptoms.

- Taking ten to twenty drops of tincture of dandelion root three times a day with meals will usually eliminate water retention. Alternatively, drink three cups of dandelion root tea a day made with one teaspoon of dandelion root in a cup of boiling water.
- St John's Wort (*Hypericum perforatum*) rubbed on to sore breasts relieves pain thanks to its action on nerve endings.
- Tincture of yellow dock root (*Rumex crispus*) – five to ten drops two or three times a day – can help to counter indigestion, constipation and intestinal gas.
- Sage (*Salvia officinalis*) is rich in phyto-hormones. Drinking sage tea or taking tincture of sage (ten to twenty drops three times a day) can help to counteract PMS.

Diet

Excessive consumption of animal fat increases oestrogen levels and decreases progesterone levels thus contributing to PMS. Studies show that PMS patients consume 62 per cent more refined carbohydrates, 275 per cent more refined sugar, 78 per cent more salt, 79 per cent more dairy products, 53 per cent less iron, 77 per cent less manganese and 52 per cent less zinc than do women without PMS. They are also lower in B complex vitamins than normal women. Initiating the dietary changes suggested in previous chapters can be instrumental in eliminating PMS. Dr Tori Hudson, Academic Dean at the Natural College of Naturopathic Medicine in Portland, Oregon, recommends that a diet to protect women from PMS should include fresh vegetables and fruit, whole grains, legumes, nuts, seeds and fish, and exclude refined sugars, large quantities of protein, dairy products, free fats, salt, caffeine, and tobacco. Another major item to avoid at all costs is junk fats: salad oils, margarines, and convenience foods filled with processed trans fatty acids. These, more than any single dietary item, interfere with hormonal functions.

Using a simple detoxification programme based on fresh foods every four to six months, such as the Miso Detox and Rebuild (see Step Three) can clear away the accumulation of wastes that interferes with the proper functioning of the reproductive system. Even a day or two a month on miso broth and seaweed in the week before a period helps to cleanse the body and rebalance the system.

Nutritional Support

No nutritional supplement is going to replace a proper diet and lifestyle which supports your energy and is a reflection of the value you place on yourself. However, certain supplements, especially magnesium, zinc, vitamin B_6 and the other B vitamins, can help to alleviate PMS and should be considered. In an uncontrolled study where women with PMS were given a multivitamin and mineral supplement containing high doses of magnesium and vitamin B_6, seventy per cent showed a reduction in symptoms.

- Magnesium is an essential catalyst in many enzyme reactions, particularly those involved in energy production and sugar metabolism. A deficiency in magnesium appears to be a strong factor in the development of PMS. Magnesium levels are significantly lower in PMS sufferers than in other women. Low magnesium often produces symptoms of aches and pains as well as nervousness, lowered immunity, breast pain and weight gain. Take 400–800 mg chelated magnesium a day in split doses.
- Vitamin B complex deficiencies result in depressed liver functions. Much PMS develops out of an excess of oestrogens in the blood caused by the liver's inability to clear them from the system. Take a vitamin B complex supplement, 25–50 mg a day.
- Zinc deficiencies are common in women who have taken synthetic hormones in the contraceptive pill and HRT.

Coffee and tea also interfere with zinc absorption. Take 18–22 mg chelated zinc or zinc picolinate a day, preferably at night.

- Studies show that women given vitamin E supplements experience significant improvement in PMS symptoms including headaches, tiredness, depression, insomnia and nervous tension. Take 200–400 iu (international units) a day.

- Beta-carotene, a precursor to vitamin A, is a safe alternative to vitamin A itself. In studies it has been shown to reduce PMS symptoms. Take 50,000 iu a day.

- Bioflavinoids – substances such as *quercetin* and *apigenin* inhibit the actions of excess oestrogen and have been shown to be useful in eliminating many symptoms of PMS. Take mixed flavinoids, 1000 mg a day.

- Essential fatty acids are necessary in order for the body to manufacture and use hormones properly. The metabolism of essential fatty acids requires adequate magnesium, vitamin C, zinc, vitamin B_6 and vitamin B_3. This is a major reason why all of these nutrients are so important in the treatment of PMS. Using borage oil, or evening primrose oil supplements which are all high in GLA, can be very helpful. Take 500 mg three to four times a day. You can also use flaxseed oil or Udo's Choice (see Resources), one or two tablespoons poured over salads or vegetables every day.

Progesterone

Underlying all pre-menstrual problems, whether primarily nutritional, emotional or stress-related in origin, is an imbalance in hormones. In most PMS the imbalance in hormones is a simple one: too much oestrogen and too little progesterone. While this is not the case for every woman, it is certainly true in the vast majority of cases. Many of the common treatments for PMS, from the use of extra vitamin B_6 to changes in diet – actually work because they influence hormone balance.

The water retention which occurs near a menstrual period is not simple oedema. Water actually gets blocked within cells. This can mean a weight gain of as much as 3.5 kilos (8 lb) over the ten days just before a period. Using a progesterone cream for three months from day twelve to day twenty-six or seven of the menstrual cycle will almost invariably cure this problem. John Lee suggests that, after using the cream for several weeks, women weigh themselves during the time of the month when they formerly experienced the waterlogging. 'When a woman sees that the oedema is now gone,' says Lee, 'it proves to her that the progesterone is working.' After using progesterone cream, Lee's patients report that they feel much better, that they feel they have a handle on their life again, they can get on with things without the disturbing effects of their PMS. 'Not all PMS is due to progesterone deficiency or oestrogen-dominance,' says Lee, 'but a wide proportion of PMS women have oestrogen-dominance and are helped by progesterone.'

John Lee's Protocols for PMS

John Lee recommends using a 50-gram (2-oz) jar of progesterone cream in the ten days just before your period. With experience many women discover that the progesterone dose can be applied so that it produces a crescendo effect in the four or five days immediately before menstruation begins. In fact, some women use drops of progesterone oil under the tongue during the last four or five days in addition to the progesterone cream. Others apply extra cream several times a day just before a period. 'The important thing to remember about dose,' says Lee, 'is that the right dose of progesterone for any particular woman is the dose that works.' To achieve the crescendo dose, Lee suggests that a woman should use a full 50-gram (2-oz) jar of the progesterone cream in ten or twelve days, between days fourteen and twenty-six or days twelve and twenty-eight, aiming to have finished the jar two days before her period. In the last five days she should add four drops of progesterone oil under the tongue each day. Taking progesterone oil is a little tricky, as it has to be held under the tongue for three to five minutes to allow it to be properly absorbed through the mucous membranes of the mouth. Learning to hold the oil there for long enough without swallowing may take practice.

Step Seven
Chill Out

ONE DAY – an ordinary day like any other – almost imperceptibly at first you sense something strange happening in your body. A tiny flutter of heat begins to rise and sweep up your torso, neck and head. The feeling passes almost as quickly as it came, and you find you are feeling just a bit chilled. Or maybe one night at 3 a.m. you awaken to find yourself drenched in sweat for no reason. 'Am I ill?' you ask, making a quick check through your body only to find that no, you do not feel ill. 'Then what on earth is happening?' Hot flushes are the most common herald of menopause – they are virtually synonymous with it. An adjunct to hot flushes are night sweats: women wake up drenched in sweat, so much so that they may need to change the sheets as well as their nightclothes. Both night sweats and hot flushes can be disconcerting, even frightening. Step Seven looks at what they are and how to deal with them.

Cross Currents

Although a lot can be said about hot flushes, only two things are absolutely essential to know: first, they are completely harmless; second, out of a long list of symptoms attributed to menopause, hot flushes are virtually the only ones that are genuinely linked to it. This was established by research carried out at Oxford and reported in *The British Medical Journal*. The study compared mid-life women with mid-life men in an attempt to find out which of women's complaints were menopausal. Scientists reported that among those symptoms generally lumped together under the menopausal label –

including aches in joints, migraine and depression – only hot flushes show a direct relationship to menopause itself. Another interesting study carried out in Canada by Pat Kaufert found that despite all the fuss about hot flushes, most women still look upon them as normal and believe they don't detract from general good health.

Menopausal women are not the only people who get hot flushes. They can also occur during pregnancy as well as just after giving birth. Men too will experience them after any kind of rapid withdrawal of sex hormones. Women of all ages get them especially strongly when their ovaries are removed surgically, as do men when their testicles are removed. At the time of menopause, thinner women tend to experience more drastic alterations in their oestrogen levels and are therefore more likely than their bigger sisters to experience strong hot flushes.

No Great Matter

During a hot flush blood rushes into the capillaries, the pulse rate rises and skin temperature goes up. Hot flushes do not appear to affect blood pressure, but they are often followed by a chilled feeling. Both oestrogen and progesterone play a role in bodily temperature regulation. In most women hot flushes are at their most intense during the last year or so before the end of menstruation and during the first year or so afterwards. What do they feel like? This differs almost as much as individual women do. Generally there is a flush of heat which sweeps over your torso, neck and head. You feel the need to take off your sweater or jacket for a few minutes, but will probably want to put it back on again soon, because the body's reaction to the flush can leave you feeling a little chilled. Hot flushes may make your skin go red or even blotchy. Sometimes they are followed by perspiration, which can range from a little glow to a torrent of water. Usually a hot flush lasts from a few seconds to a couple of minutes. Very rarely they can last as long as fifteen minutes or more.

How often they happen is also highly individual. A very few women seem to experience hot flushes – at least for a short period of their life – every hour or two. Others get them only at certain times of the day or night. Some women can report up to thirty hot flushes a day while most experience only one or two. A few women don't get them at all. The prevalence of hot flushes is virtually 100 per cent among women who have gone through an artificially induced menopause as a result of surgery. After surgery, symptoms are much more intense and the flushes come much more frequently than they did before. Factors that predispose women to hot flushes have been little studied. What is known is that there is no correlation between hot flushes and socio-economic groups, employment status, or medical status. Neither is the incidence of hot flushes related to the age at which a woman began to menstruate, to her age at menopause, or to the number of children that she has had. The one factor that does appear to correlate with hot flushes is that women who get them tend to have a lower body weight than women who do not.

The Real Thing

Research has shown that oestrogen levels tend to be lower in pre-menopausal women with hot flushes than in those without. However, it is quite clear that low oestrogen levels, although they are continually blamed for causing hot flushes, are by no means the single factor in their production. It is the sudden drop in oestrogen which is important. Once the body becomes accustomed to lower levels of oestrogen, hot flushes gradually diminish, as a rule. Sometimes low oestrogen is not involved in hot flushes at all. A small number of women go into menopause in their teens and twenties as a result of genetic abnormalities. These women experience hot flushes only if they take supplementary oestrogen in HRT for a time and then stop. Many post-menopausal women with low oestrogen levels never have hot flushes. Before puberty, when oestrogen levels are very low, girls do not have hot flushes. On the other hand, hot flushes are reported by some women during pregnancy or immediately after giving birth, when oestrogen levels are high.

Certain factors are known to contribute to the incidence of hot flushes. If you are troubled by their intensity you might like to avoid cigarette smoking, caffeine and hot, spicy foods. An overactive thyroid can cause hot flushes, as can untreated diabetes. According to Dr Ellen Grant, author of the courageous book *Sexual Chemistry*, hot flushes may be the result of allergic reactions, particularly to foods or chemicals in the environment. The high levels of steroid hormones used in HRT tend to suppress certain functions in the body such as those which are connected with allergies and with the body's attempt to detoxify itself. Dr Grant believes that when oestrogen decreases rapidly in a menopausal woman or in someone who has been taking extra hormones, the underlying allergy or toxicity which was being masked by the hormones comes to the surface. Hot flushes can be the result. At the Charing Cross Hospital Migraine Clinic, Grant requested that her patients explore for themselves which foods gave them reactions such as migraine, headaches and raised blood pressure as well as hot flushes. She found that when an offending food such as milk, wheat, cheese, chocolate or oranges is removed from the diet, hot flushes will diminish, and even cease altogether.

Common Treatment

The standard medical treatment for hot flushes is oestrogen. If you decide to go on oestrogen for a few years 'to get you through the rough patch', what you are not told is that when you come off – three years down the line or twenty – your hot flushes are very likely to return in force. Extra oestrogen does not 'cure' hot flushes. It only masks them for a while. In any case, there is nothing to 'cure'. Hot flushes are not a symptom of disease. They are a normal bodily change associated with the transition between the menstrual years and menopause. Women who have learnt to fear menopause – particularly professional women – sometimes dread a hot flush coming over them during a business meeting, for example, and betraying their menopausal condition. Most hot flushes happen without anybody knowing except the woman herself. Women always think they are more evident to the outside world than they are. And even if they were obvious, so what? Why should a woman even tacitly buy into the general consensus that menopause – like the swollen belly of pregnancy in days gone by – is something disgraceful, to be hidden.

Look Within

According to Eastern religions and traditional medicine, a hot flush is a rapid release of kundalini energy, creative energy which is said to rise up the spine, refining the nervous system and activating the energy centres in the body. When the kundalini fire rises in a menopausal woman she becomes capable of powerful healing, wisdom and peace-keeping – the traditional role of the postmenopausal woman or 'crone' in many societies. It can be useful to view hot flushes from this point of view. It is often helpful to see them as your own creative energy finally being made available to use as you choose, instead of being channelled into carrying and raising children. I have worked with many groups of menopausal women by approaching hot flushes in this way. We have looked at them not as something to be feared or concealed but rather as a sign that a woman's individual spirit, often long ignored, is demanding attention. Once you take notice, hot flushes can offer the most phenomenal energy to use for whatever you most want in life.

Self-help

Some of the most interesting research into the incidence of hot flushes has involved observations of the effect of diet and cultural attitudes. In Indonesia and Japan women experience very few hot flushes, particularly compared with women in Western societies. Mayan Indians in Mexico report no symptoms at the approach of menopause other than the menstrual cycle becoming irregular. It would appear that there are significant dietary differences operating here. For example, Japanese women eat lots of soya products which contain high levels of plant hormones and have few symptoms of menopause.

Certain plants are high in oestrogen-like hormones – beetroot, potato root, parsley root, and yeast, for instance, all of which contain 70–80 picograms of these natural phytohormones per 100 grams. Natural unheated honey contains 40–600 iu per kilo, while dry sage boasts 6000 iu per kilo. Clover is similarly high in phyto-hormones, as are alfalfa, fennel, celery, anise and liquorice. A diet which includes these and is high in other hormone-rich foods (see Step Five) should supply a much higher level of protective natural hormones and do much to alleviate hot flushes. Herbs are also very helpful:

- *Sage* Make an infusion of one teaspoon of the dried leaves in a cup of water, allow it to steep for ten minutes, then drink one tablespoon of the tea one to eight times a day. Or you can take ten to twenty-five drops of tincture of sage every day. Use sage liberally in your cooking too.
- *Motherwort* It does not make a nice-tasting tea, so I prefer to take motherwort as a tincture. Take ten to twenty-five drops of tincture every two to six hours.
- *Chastetree* Take one capsule of powdered berries three to four times a day, or fifteen drops to one teaspoonful of the tincture one to three times a day.
- *Dong Quai* Make an infusion of a teaspoon of the dried root in a cup of boiling water and drink once a day. Or take fifteen to thirty drops of tincture one to three times a day.

I Lie Burning

The long traditions of European natural medicine views hot flushes as the body's way of detoxifying itself and enhancing immunity. Recent research shows that even a slight rise in body temperature can be instrumental in doing both. A few months before she died, I interviewed Dr Dagmar Leichti von Brasch (see page 103), director of the world-famous Bircher

Benner clinic. When I asked her to tell me about hot flushes from the point of view of natural medicine, she explained that, like night sweats, they have always been considered the means by which a woman's body deep-cleanses itself and refines itself for new physical and spiritual tasks. I also questioned Leichti at some length about her own experience of menopause and about the experiences of the thousands of mid-life women patients she had cared for during more than half a century of practising medicine. She said that she believed hot flushes and waking in the night in sweat can be important events in a woman's spiritual life. 'They stop us from carrying on "as normal", which women are so apt to do – fulfilling their social roles. They demand that we pay attention to our bodies and to our lives,' said Dr Leichti. 'This is exactly what menopausal women are supposed to do.'

A vibrant and healthy woman, Leichti ran the clinic in Zurich single-handed while fulfilling her role as wife and mother. She had the same experience during her menopause that so many peri-menopausal and menopausal women have: waking up in the wee hours of the morning for no apparent reason. This often occurs between 2 a.m. and 3 a.m. She told me she would find herself flooded in tears of the deepest sorrow. Having tried to go back to sleep, without success, she would lie in bed night after night with tears streaming down her face. For a very long while Leichti could not work out why she felt so sad, especially since every morning she would rise and go about her duties at the clinic feeling perfectly normal. Finally, after several months of this she decided that instead of remaining in bed she would get up and go to her study to write down what she felt. 'Before long,' she told me, 'I realised that I had begun to tap into new ideas which were exciting, to sense new possibilities and to see the world in new ways. It was during those early morning hours that I dreamed new dreams about my future.' Afterwards, when Leichti spoke with other women who had had similar experiences – waking in fear or grief, anger or frustration – she found that if they simply allowed themselves to feel whatever feelings arose, they discovered hidden great wells of energy, creativity and insight.

Living In Time

I too have had the experience of waking up night after night. I would awaken like clockwork at 3 a.m. and lie in bed in a state that can only be described as a mixture of terror and frustration. I could never go back to sleep. I kept feeling that I wanted to get up and do something. I had a strange desire to leave my house and walk barefoot down the path through the woods to the sea. Then the fear would arise, the fear of doing something so unconventional, something I was not used to doing. Perhaps it was a fear of madness. At that time I had no idea that what I was feeling was connected with my coming menopause. I was menstruating normally and had only begun to have the odd hot flush, which did not worry me or seem particularly strange, since it was very much how I feel during vigorous exercise. Later on, just at the point when my periods stopped, I began to get up in the night. I would go into my studio, turn on the lights and work. At that time I was finishing my first novel. Then, sometimes after two or three hours, I would climb back into bed and sleep for an hour before getting up to send my youngest son off to school. I relished that hour. Such a deep and blissful sleep came then, a sleep full of dreams and new visions. Later I was to discover, as Dr Leichti had, that the work I did during my night vigils was the most creative work I had ever done. Since then, having spoken with dozens of women who report similar experiences, I have come to believe that hot flushes, night sweats, night wakings and many of the other events associated with menopause often bring to the surface parts of ourselves which we have long ignored. In Leichti's case it was buried sorrow, in my own it was profound frustration about my work and a great deal of fear, in other women it can be resentment or grief, sadness or even wonder and a new kind of joy. For all of us, hidden beneath these feelings and night events are new ways of looking at the world, even whole new lives, just waiting to be noticed. We should stop and listen instead of trying to batten down the hatches and carry on 'as normal'.

Never Come Morning

Insomnia is one of women's greatest fears. Eight times more women than men report sleep difficulties to their doctors. Apart from the motherhood-induced insomnia which comes from having to feed a baby, if ever you are going to have trouble sleeping it is most likely to be either during the peri-menopausal years just before your periods stop or much later on, in your seventies and eighties. People sleep less as they get older for a number of reasons, not the least of which is a decrease in the production of a substance called melatonin that regulates the body's circadian rhythms. Hot flushes and night sweats can interfere with sleep too, but often simply dealing with the feelings you wake up with is enough to make you sleep blissfully through the night. Sleep patterns vary tremendously from person to person. Some women need only four or five hours a night, while others need eight or nine. Short sleepers are often more outgoing, contented and lively than their long-sleeping sisters who may get as much as ten hours a night. Studies show that long sleepers tend to worry more, and be more introverted and anxious. How much sleep you need can change depending on your life circumstances, too. When you are pregnant, eat less wholesome foods, or are under stress or ill you may need more sleep. You also need more sleep when you gain weight. When losing weight, or during a detoxification regime, you will often sleep less, to no ill effect.

Common Treatment

Nevertheless, when sleeplessness becomes chronic it can leave you feeling exhausted, hopeless and washed out, in which case something needs to be done about it. Sleeping pills are not the answer. Their side-effects include digestive problems, poor concentration, disorders of the blood and respiration, high blood pressure, liver and kidney troubles, problems with vision, depression, dizziness, confusion and damage to the central nervous system. Taking them can even lead to worse insomnia. There are better ways.

Look Within

One of the most wonderful experiences for a menopausal woman is that of letting go of all time constraints and simply freewheeling. If you can manage it, take a weekend or even a week away from all responsibility either by staying at home alone or by going on a retreat so you can sleep whenever you like. Freed from the bonds of time, you can nap at any time of the day or night and heed any creative impulses that arise. Forget your watch, don't watch television or listen to the radio. See what it is like to live without the restrictions of time. It can have a remarkable effect on your creativity, and eliminate your anxiety about not sleeping as much as you think you should.

A Breath of Medicine

When sleeplessness arises out of anxiety or brings worries in its wake, it can be useful to shift the focus of your energy towards the breath, using one of the most simple yet powerful techniques I know. Practise it first when you are relaxed. Call on it during sleepless nights to transform your anxious energy into calm and at any time during the day when you feel worried or a sense of panic overcomes you.

Sitting straight in a chair or on a cushion on the floor with your legs crossed – once you get the hang of it you can do this exercise lying down as well – place the tip of your tongue on the ridge on your palate just behind your front teeth. Keep it there during the whole of the exercise. Breathe out completely through your mouth, pursing your lips a bit if necessary, and letting the air move out around your tongue (it makes a soft whooshing sound). Now you are ready to begin.

- Close your mouth and silently inhale through the nose to a count of four.
- Hold your breath to a count of seven.
- Now exhale fully through your mouth again, making a whooshing sound as you do so, to a count of eight.
- Repeat the whole sequence four times.

The in-breath is taken silently through the nose with the mouth closed, and the out-breath, which takes twice as long, is made through the slightly opened mouth. How much time you spend on each phase of the breath is up to you. To begin with, it is likely to be faster and later on, when you have used the exercise a lot, it is likely to slow down a great deal. This really does not matter. What is important is that you maintain the same 4:7:8 ratio.

This marvellous exercise brings about an instantaneous shift of consciousness after only four breaths. Use it whenever you feel anxious or stressed. After you have learned it and used it for a few weeks, you can extend from four to eight breaths for even deeper calming effects. Don't try this until you know the sequence well, as it might make you slightly light-headed.

Self-help

There are some excellent herb helpers for sleeplessness. Each has its own character and some will work better for you than others. Here are my favourites:

- **Valerian** comes from the root of the plant *Valeriana officinalis,* which was the primary herbal sedative used on both sides of the Atlantic before the advent of barbiturate sleeping pills. It is a safe and well-tested herbal remedy with a smell like dirty old socks (the smell drives some people's cats wild). Don't let that put you off: valerian is a powerful and useful tool for inducing safe sleep, more potent than most of the other natural tranquillisers, such as hops, skull-cap and camomile. You can take valerian in a couple of ways, but I like the tincture best: ten to twenty drops before bedtime in a little water or in the middle of the night when you wake. Alternatively, you can use a couple of capsules of the dried root. Valerian in lower doses is also useful when your nerves feel 'shot' during the day. Very occasionally valerian can cause a little sense of hangover in the morning. If this happens to you, either cut down on the dose or try another remedy. It can be a good idea to change remedies every so often; if your body becomes accustomed to a remedy, its effect may be lessened.

- **Passionflower** (*Passiflora incarnata*), also known as Maypops, is a climbing plant that boasts magnificent white flowers with a purple centre. It has a wonderful sedative and mildly narcotic effect on the body. Passionflower is most useful for women who frequently suffer from nervous tension, and is particularly helpful before and around the time of menopause, when hormones can fluctuate wildly and nerves may be on edge. It is also useful for relieving pain, thanks to its mild pain-killing and anti-spasmodic qualities (which have been well demonstrated in laboratory and clinical tests) and for pre-menstrual tension. Not as strong as valerian in its actions, it is more calming than sedating, and as such is a great alternative to tranquilliser drugs. Use ten to twenty drops of the tincture or the liquid extract in water. Alternatively, take two capsules of the dried extract up to four times a day as needed. Whereas valerian tends to be taken at night, just before bed, the best results from passionflower often come from taking it two to four times a day; it will calm nerves and make everything easier and less stressful.

- **Camomile Tea** (*Matricaria chamomilla*). One of the nine herbs sacred to the Anglo-Saxon god Wotan, camomile was also much loved by the Romans. Its name *Matricaria* is derived either from the Latin word *mater*, meaning 'mother', or from *matrix* meaning 'womb'. It has for thousands of years been used as a woman's herb against painful menstruation, to calm anxiety and aid sleep, and even to help build strong bones, since it contains a form of readily absorbed calcium. Camomile is also a uterine tonic, a property that has been scientifically evaluated. It boasts many other therapeutic properties, such as being anti-bacterial in its actions and good for skin. The easiest way to take camomile is in the form of a tea. Infuse a teaspoon of the dried flowers in hot water before bed or whenever you need to relax. Camomile works particularly well when taken together with passionflower.

- **Hops** (*Humulus lupulus*). The flowers from this British herb are often used together with other remedies to treat everything from indigestion to frazzled nerves. Like valerian, hops have a pronounced sedative effect, but they are milder. Unlike valerian, they smell sweet and can be used without concern for side-effects. You can use hops in the form of a tincture but by far the best way for sleep – particularly good for women who wake in the middle of the night and have trouble going back to sleep – is to drink hop tea. Make it before going to bed by steeping a tea-spoon of the flowers for ten minutes in hot water, then strain and allow to cool. Drink it sweetened with honey if you like. Leave a cup of hop tea beside your bed so you can drink it when you wake in the night. Also wonderful is a little pillow stuffed with dried hop blossoms which you put under your neck when you go to bed or if you wake up.

- **Oatstraw** (*Avena sativa*). The straw from oats can restore energy when nerves have been frayed, counteract insomnia, ease night sweats, calm anxiety and even relieve headache. Stuff a little pillow with oat hulls or infuse a tea-spoon of them in hot water and keep the tea beside your bed at night in case you need it.

Hormone Magic: Melatonin

During the hours of darkness the pineal gland in the centre of the brain secretes a hormone called melatonin, acting in direct response to the amount of sunlight we were exposed to during the preceding days. It is a deficiency in melatonin production which produces the now widely publicised

Seasonal Affective Disorder, or SAD, causing depression in some people during long, dark winters. The whole melatonin issue is a particularly important one for menopausal women. The production of melatonin tends to drop as the body gets older. Many age-researchers now believe that supplements of melatonin can combat ageing. Melatonin shortens the time that a woman stays awake when she wakes in the night, and reduces the number of times she wakes up. It increases daytime alertness and energy levels as well. The dose generally recommended is between three and fifteen milligrams, preferably taken on an empty stomach an hour before bed, although some people seem to need more. Melatonin is one of those compounds which, although it has often been given in much higher doses – between forty and eighty milligrams – appears to be more effective for many women in low doses.

Sleep Rituals

When it comes to getting ready for sleep at night, the body loves routines. They foster relaxation and let it know what to expect.

- Make bedtime and rising time as regular as possible and go through the same routine each evening of locking the front door, opening the bedroom window, reading a book, or whatever suits you.
- Take plenty of aerobic exercise each week, preferably out of doors. Experiment with exercising at different times of the day to see which is best for relaxing you and making you ready for sleep at night.
- Stay awake: don't start any new activities late in the day and avoid taking a nap in the evening or late afternoon.
- Eat Early. Don't eat dinner late in the evening – the earlier the better. Make it the smallest meal of the day and avoid snacks after dinner, since they can interfere with sleep. Everybody sleeps better on an empty stomach, despite what all the hot-drink manufacturers would have you believe.
- At bedtime, soak in a lukewarm (not hot) bath for thirty minutes, topping up with hot water to maintain the

temperature at just blood heat. Blot your skin dry without friction and go straight to bed, moving slowly. This can be a great thing to do if you wake up in the middle of the night, too. Use a candle instead of turning on the light and let yourself relax as you probably never can during the day, when a telephone could ring or someone might demand something from you.

- Sleep alone: insist on sleeping in a room by yourself if you prefer. Many women stay in the same bed with their mate night after night, year after year out of habit, from insecurity, or for fear of upsetting the boat should they voice a need for solitude at night. Just as it is every woman's right to refuse to have sex with a partner, it is her right to sleep alone when she wishes. If you never insist upon your own night space, however, it is very unlikely ever to be offered to you.

- Drink plenty of water during the day. Sleep is induced by the brain and brain cells need adequate hydration, both to stay awake during the daylight hours and to trigger the dreamy relaxation that brings on sleep. Hardly anyone drinks as much water as they profitably could. I discovered this a couple of years ago and now regularly consume at least two litres of mineral water a day in addition to what-ever other drinks I may have.

- Cut out all stimulants, such as coffee, tea, and colas. These can prevent a good night's sleep when they are in your sys-tem, even if you have taken them many hours before bed-time.

- Give thanks. Count your blessings. This is an old-fashioned idea, but it is a true key to deep relaxation and blissful sleep. Each night, as you turn out the light, think of six things to be thankful for, regardless of your physical or emotional state or how difficult your life may be at any time. This gradually trains the mind to dwell on pleasur-able themes even when you are awake. It can improve the quality of your dreams, too.

Build Bones

OSTEOPOROSIS is a terrible disease. A progressive loss of minerals, bone mass and bone density, it affects men as well as women and can result in fractures of the hip, shoulder, ribs, vertebrae, forearm or wrist. Statistically, bone loss in women begins several years before menopause and then gets worse afterwards, creating an ever-increasing risk of debilitating breakages. Osteoporosis is now the most common bone disorder in the West. In Britain where the incidence of the illness has increased six-fold in the past thirty years, one in three women and one in eight men now develop it. In the United States the statistics are even worse: the illness currently costs the country more than eleven billion dollars a year. Twenty-five per cent of women whose hips fracture die within two years, not always as a direct result of the fracture, but from ending up in nursing homes, where inactivity, alienation and loss of control over their lives defeat them. Today more women in the industrialised world die of fractures related to bone thinning than from cancers of the womb, cervix and breast put together. Yet this is preventable. Step Eight shows you how.

Silent Killer

Osteoporosis is not a simple disorder. And it is most certainly not another so-called oestrogen deficiency disease, as some would still have us believe. Neither is it treatable by drinking masses of milk or stuffing yourself with calcium supplements, which, surprisingly perhaps, can actually make the condition worse. Osteoporosis is an insidious illness. It develops secretly over the years until one day its presence surfaces to devastate your life. It need not.

A few facts: osteoporosis regularly occurs in men who are deficient in testosterone and in women who are deficient in progesterone. Black women have less bone loss than white women, big women less than small women and fat women less than their skinny sisters. Meat-eaters are at far greater risk of the disease than vegetarians. A high calcium intake is often regarded as essential in preventing bone thinning. Yet people in Third World countries whose daily intake of calcium is less than half our own have a very low incidence of the disease. More users of prescription drugs develop osteoporosis than people who do not take medication. And couch potatoes are far more prone to the condition than women who get regular exercise – particularly weight-bearing exercise. Osteoporosis is a complex condition. To prevent it you need to understand it. Despite all the fear-mongering surrounding the disease, the truth is that once you know your stuff there are actions you can take not only to halt bone loss if it has begun but even to reverse it – no matter what your age.

Living Bone

Bones may seem like tough, inanimate objects, but they are not. They are actually living tissue, always changing and growing. Your bones are constantly being renewed – at a surprising rate. This is what makes it possible for breaks to mend and for a child's body to grow taller. When you are born, growth hormone stimulates your bones to grow at a rate that in general matches the rate at which the rest of your body is growing. After puberty the hormones of the ovaries take over. It becomes the job of oestrogen to slow down or moderate the rate at which old bone is broken down. Meanwhile proges-terone encourages the manufacture of new bone. If these two processes are in complete harmony – working at the same rate – your skeleton will maintain the same strength. When new bone formation exceeds breakdown, your bones will grow denser and stronger. If breakdown begins to overtake new bone production, osteoporosis develops. Think of bones as the fibres that make up a scarf or shawl, fibres that are knitted together with little spaces in between. When osteoporosis occurs, not only have the fibres become finer, you actually have fewer of them. In effect, you have lost a number of bone strands and each strand that is left has become thinner. Under the microscope – sometimes even with the naked eye – you can see there are spaces in bone which make it look spongy or porous. Osteoporosis comes from *osteon*, meaning 'bone', and *porosus*, meaning 'full of pores'.

Personal Pacman

The ability of bones to break down and reform is determined by a process called remodelling, which relies on two very special kinds of cells. The first are called *osteoclasts*. If you have ever played the videogame *Pacman* you will find it easy to understand how they work. It is the job of the oestrogen-regulated osteoclasts to travel through your bone tissue like Pacman, seek out old bone and gobble it up or dissolve it away – the proper term is *resorb* it – in order to leave spaces to make way for new bone. After the osteoclasts have done their work, along come the other kind of bone cells: the *osteoblasts*. These cells, whose activity is regulated by progesterone, are drawn to the same sites. They make their way into these spaces and start creating new bone.

When you are growing up, the action of your osteoblasts is greater than that of the osteoclasts and more bone is created than is destroyed. Around puberty the activity of osteoclasts and osteoblasts is about even. Later on, however, the balance can shift in favour of the bone-eating osteoclasts, while osteoblast activity declines. It is now that osteoporosis first takes hold. More spaces are appearing than are being filled. If this goes on for a long time, too many minerals can be lost. Bone becomes less hard and less dense until at last it is finely honeycombed and highly susceptible to breakage. It is during the five to eight years before menopause that women are most vulnerable to bone loss. Insufficient progesterone leads to insufficient osteoblast activity. Without enough progesterone the osteoblasts are unable to produce new bone properly, so more bone is resorbed than built and osteoporosis sets in. Statistically, bone mass in healthy women reaches a peak in their early thirties. After that, osteoclast activity tends to increase, while osteoblast activity gradually declines. To prevent, stop and reverse bone loss you need to do two things: get your hormone balance right and change your lifestyle.

Hormone Connections

It was pressure from hundreds of women with osteoporosis that triggered Dr John Lee's experiments with progesterone. He asked himself, since oestrogen is still produced by post-menopausal women, 'Could progesterone alone be enough to prevent and/or reverse osteoporosis?' Lee began to test out his hypothesis with women who had post-menopausal osteo-porosis, using progesterone cream rubbed on to the skin, together with a programme of dietary changes, vitamin and mineral supplements, and modest exercise. Some of his patients were also given very small doses of oestrogen, particularly if they suffered from vaginal dryness. Lee care-fully monitored his results, keeping records for more than ten years. When at last they were published, his findings turned out to be nothing short of revolutionary. He had been able to accomplish the impossible. The natural progesterone cream halted bone loss, whether or not the women taking it had been given oestrogen as well. Remarkably, his patients showed an improvement of approximately fifteen per cent in bone mineral density over a three-year period. Even more surprisingly, the women with the worst bones improved fastest. Some of them showed much greater than average improvement – a thirty to forty per cent increase in bone over the three-year period was not uncommon. Those women whose bone density was fairly good when the experiment began improved more slowly, until finally each woman – no matter what condition her bones had been in at the start of the study – reached her optimum bone density and then maintained it. Although such successes are great news, do not be tempted to think that all you need to do to prevent osteoporosis is to rub on progesterone cream every day and then sit back munching on junk food, certain that all will be well. The trouble is, it just doesn't work that way. What you eat and how you live are equally important.

Stress Your Body

All any woman needs to maintain good, strong, dense, well-mineralised bones is a good balance between the activity of her osteoblasts and her osteoclasts. A woman in the Western world living a sedentary life and eating convenience foods will find this virtually impossible. During a woman's menstruating years her body's ability to build new bone often declines as a result of inadequate minerals or vitamins in her diet. This is virtually always a problem if she lives on the standard Western fare or if she goes on and off slimming diets. The highly processed foods on which most of us live these days are not only deficient in zinc, magnesium and vitamin C – all of which are essential for good bone remodelling – they are very low in little-known micronutrients such as silica and boron which also play important roles in good bone formation. Eating too much meat can lead to bone loss. A high-protein diet draws calcium out of the bones like a sponge, pouring it into the bloodstream, from where it gets excreted through the urine. Many forms of purified protein regularly used in slimmers' meal-replacement drinks cause calcium loss too, especially when used regularly. In fact, crash dieting of any kind is a common contributor to bone thinning in women. So is taking in too much phosphorous by drinking soft drinks such as diet colas or eating processed meats. Excess phosphorous leaches calcium, destroying bone strength and density. Three other things are also associated with rapid bone loss: cigarette smoking, inadequate exercise, and excess alcohol. As far as bone building is concerned, every woman regardless of age needs regular weight-bearing exercise. While cycling, running, skipping, walking and swimming are great for your heart and lungs, they do little to stress your skeleton. For that you need weight training. Your bones need to be physically stressed if you are to maintain good bone strength.

Calcium Connections

In every case of osteoporosis calcium loss from the bones lies at the core of the problem. Calcium is the most abundant mineral in your body. It is vital for strong bones. About ninety-nine per cent of the calcium in your body is deposited in your bones and teeth, although the remaining one per cent has some very important jobs to do too. It helps to regulate nerve and muscle contraction, for instance. Calcium also enables your body to use iron properly and activate a number of important enzymes that help to regulate the passage of nutrients into and out of the cells. Finally, calcium is frequently called on – and called forth from bones – to balance the pH of your blood, making it more alkaline when it has become too acid from long-term stress, eating a lot of meat, or drinking a lot of coffee.

In case all this makes you think you must rush out and buy a bottle of calcium pills, think again. Despite all the vitamin manufacturers currently pushing calcium supplements, research shows that taking calcium supplements is of little help in preventing osteoporosis. In fact, it may even make the problem worse. Taking higher doses of calcium supplements can contribute to kidney stones and interfere with your body's use of zinc and magnesium, both of which play central roles in building strong bones. The best way to get your calcium is to eat the right kind of foods, particularly green, leafy vegetables and sea plants, which are loaded with calcium in a form that is easy for the body to assimilate.

Forget the Milk

We have been led to believe that all you need for strong bones is to consume lots of calcium either by popping pills or drinking masses of milk. Millions have been spent to propagate this fantasy. Yet after three generations of milk promotion osteoporosis has now reached epidemic proportions in the West, while in countries where milk is not drunk it hardly exists. Milk and milk products have an extremely negative effect on a woman's health in general. Experiment by leaving all milk products out of your diet for three weeks and you are likely to find your looks and energy levels will certainly be transformed for the better. This can be difficult, since in one form or another milk finds its way into most convenience foods – even bread.

As we grow up our bodies gradually lose the ability to produce the enzyme which digests the sugar in milk. This creates what is known as a *lactose intolerance*. Studies show that three out of every four adults in the United States have some degree of lactose intolerance. They are unable to digest milk properly. If they include dairy foods in their diet, their energy levels may be lowered, their bodies may produce more mucus in an immune reaction, and they may fall prey to food sensitivity reactions such as mood swings or depression as well as aches and pains. Milk is the most common food allergen in the Western world. Wheat follows close behind it. Yet milk is found just about everywhere – in cheese, cream, foods with cream sauces, yoghurt, ice-cream, breads, and other commercially prepared food products. Far from turning to milk as a source of calcium, most women who value wellbeing and good looks would be better off banning milk from their diet altogether. This includes anything that might contain milk products such as milk solids, sodium caseinate, sodium lactate, milk fats, whey, or lactose too.

We are repeatedly told that the best source of calcium is milk or milk products, but rarely ask where the calcium in milk comes from in the first place. Cows get calcium from eating green foods – grass, silage, herbs and plants – which can take the calcium from the soil and turn it into a form available for absorption by animals. Beetroot tops, Chinese leaves, rocket, lettuce, seaweeds, herbs and broad-leafed green vegetables are all excellent sources of calcium. A cup of any of these vegetables supplies as much calcium as a cup of milk. Such foods provide a type of calcium that is easily used by the body, along with other important minerals and trace elements from such foods, and causes none of the negative side-effects of using milk products. Include plenty of leafy green vegetables in your meals and you need never give calcium another thought.

The reason why taking calcium supplements or drinking masses of milk has very little effect in halting – and none at all in reversing – osteoporosis is because it is usually not an absence of calcium in the body which is the problem so much as a disorder in the way calcium is absorbed.

A Delicate Process

The absorption of calcium in general tends to be highly inefficient. Only somewhere between twenty and thirty per cent of the calcium you take in through your food will actually be absorbed. The rest gets filtered through your blood and then flushed out of your body. When you are growing rapidly or when you place stress on your bones doing weight-bearing exercise, your absorption of calcium is increased. In fact, the smaller the supply of calcium available from your food and the greater the need your body has for this mineral, the more efficient calcium absorption becomes. The opposite is also true. When large quantities of calcium are available – say if a woman has been drinking a lot of milk or has taken masses of calcium supplements – the absorption of calcium is markedly decreased.

For proper absorption, calcium needs enough acid in the digestive tract. As people get older the hydrochloric acid content of the stomach tends to decrease. With this decrease comes a further decrease in the body's ability to assimilate calcium. Calcium absorption also requires adequate vitamin D, which regulates the level of calcium in the blood, and the mineral phosphorus, which is essential to build bone. But if either calcium or phosphorus are taken in excess – the typical Western diet of convenience foods, with cured meats, colas and diet drinks is very high in phosphorus – then neither element can be used properly and bone loss increases.

Once you begin to sense the enormous complexity and synergy involved in the absorption and use of calcium you begin to understand why it is probably best to get the calcium you need from a good diet. If you still feel you must take calcium supplements, make sure they are low dose and in a form such as calcium EAP which is more readily absorbed than the usual calcium lactate or calcium carbonate; the latter are cheap to make and form the basis of most calcium supplements. As far as oyster-shell calcium or dolomite are concerned, avoid them like the plague. They can be filled with dangerous heavy metals.

Test for Bone Loss

How do you know if you have osteoporosis? The simple answer is that you don't, because of its insidious nature. A woman may have lost a quarter of her bone by the time menopause arrives and be totally unaware of it until a fracture appears two years later. There are various medical techniques used to measure bone density. The original method was to take X-rays. Although still used in many places this is relatively useless, since X-rays cannot reliably measure bone mass loss or gain until there has been a loss of about thirty per cent. Now, with the advent of better methods, some tests can measure bone density with 96 to 98 per cent accuracy. This means they can detect a change of anything over two per cent. That change is real – you can count on it. One of these methods is *dual-energy X-ray absorptiometry* (DXA) where low-dose X-rays are used. DXA is accurate, as is *computerised tomography* (CT), but both involve radiation – especially high doses in the case of CT – which many doctors would rather not subject a woman to. Other methods, such as *single photon absorptiometry* (SPA) and *dual photon absorptiometry* (DPA) are safer, since they rely on passing light through the skin. There is, however, a simple test that you can carry out for yourself. Ask your husband or a friend to mark your height on a wall every couple of months. If your height drops as much as three millimetres in a year you need to take action, because your bones are shrinking.

Risk Factors

- Poor calcium absorption as a result of inadequate intake of vitamins and minerals including vitamin C, vitamin D, zinc and magnesium, often due to years of processed foods.
- Excess phosphorous from colas or processed meats which leaches calcium from bones.
- Excess alcohol. Alcohol renders your blood acidic and causes calcium to be leached from the bones to lower the blood's acidity.
- Physical inactivity and lack of weight-bearing exercise.
- Smoking.
- A high-protein diet. Excess protein also leaches calcium from bones, so that more is lost in the urine than is taken in through foods.
- Frequent use of diuretics, antibiotics, antacids, and drugs such as cortisone, thyroid hormones, heparin and prednisone can also disrupt the formation of good bone.
- Progesterone deficiency. This reduces the activity of osteoblast cells, leading to more old bone being broken down and less new bone being built.
- In a few women, inadequate oestrogen after menopause.

Self-help

A number of common drug treatments are advertised as useful in slowing bone loss and preventing fractures. However, most have little to offer. They include *calcitonin*, the *biphosphonates*, *anabolic steroids* and, the most commonly prescribed, *sodium fluoride*. All can have serious side-effects and none are truly effective. Be wary. There are many things you can do to help yourself.

Horsetail

Drink horsetail tea regularly. Steep one teaspoon of the dried herb in a cup of boiling water. It is rich in bone-strengthening silicon. Other herbs that go well with horsetail are sage, alfalfa, uva ursi leaves and nettle, which you can mix together and use as a bone tea regularly.

Exercise

Probably the most neglected of all the steps a woman can take to prevent and to treat osteoporosis is exercise. It needs to be weight-bearing exercise. Walking, running, cycling and aerobics might be great for general fitness but they will not get the job done when it comes to strengthening your bones because they stress only the long bones of the legs and don't supply enough load. Aerobic exercise like this will help, but it simply does not go far enough. You need weight training. The weights can be tins of beans held in each hand, dumbbells, bar bells – anything you like. Moving weights around in a way that stresses the muscles and bones all over the body is what builds strong bones. Weight training's ability to build muscle tissue and enhance the ratio of lean body mass to fat is particularly important for women as they get older since a shrinkage in lean tissue depletes the body of hormones and energy and makes the body and face look old and haggard. Weight training is easy to learn, can be done at home, and can be combined with aerobic exercise to create an unbeatable programme.

Diet

For the prevention and treatment of osteoporosis, diet is of primary importance. It should be low in fat and moderate in protein with plenty of green, leafy vegetables, no colas or processed soft drinks, and little meat or alcohol. What is wrong with excess protein? Plenty. A high-protein diet is a major cause of osteoporosis. Official World Health Organisation figures calculate that we need no more than half a gram of good-quality protein for each kilo of body weight. If you weigh 70 kilos (154 lb) that means about 35 grams (1–1 1/2 oz) of protein a day. The average Western diet serves up between 60 and 150 grams (2–5 oz) of protein a day – far more than we need. The extra protein makes blood acidic, causing the body to draw calcium out of the bones where it belongs to rebalance the excess acidity of the blood. Such a diet can result in a loss of 10 to 85 milligrams of calcium a day from the bones, regardless of calcium intake through diet or supplements. The countries with the highest consumption of protein per capita and the highest consumption of dairy products are those that have the highest incidence of hip fractures and osteoporosis. In countries where protein consumption and the consumption of dairy products are low, fractures and osteoporosis are rare.

Eat more:

- Fresh fruits. Eat them raw.
- Fresh, green, leafy vegetables such as broccoli, collards, kale, cabbage, mustard greens, Swiss chard, lambs lettuce and rocket. Eat at least fifty per cent of them raw.
- Fresh green herbs.
- Legumes such as beans, peas, lentils and chickpeas.
- Whole-grain breads, cereals, pasta and noodles, preferably two different varieties of grain a day together with one pulse. This will give you all the essential amino acids you need, even without meat. Steer clear of wheat if you suspect any sensitivity to it.

● Nuts, tofu, soya milk and other soya products including soya beans (make sure they are organic, not genetically modified) and seeds in moderation. It is not necessary to eat any animal products, but you can eat free-range eggs, fish, free-range chicken and game.

Eat less
● Dairy products (except butter in small quantities) including milk, cheese, cream and anything containing them.

Bone Makers	Bone Breakers
Adequate magnesium	Processed convenience foods and junk fats
Alfalfa and barley – high in minerals and trace elements	Diuretics and antibiotics
Boron and silicon	Crash dieting
Calcium in moderation (best from food sources)	Deficiencies in minerals and trace elements
Leafy green vegetables	Smoking
A moderate protein diet	Soft drinks including diet colas
Organically grown wholefoods	Salt
Progesterone	A high-protein diet
Sea plants and green supplements – spirulina, green algae and chlorella	A high-fat diet
Soya-based foods	Coffee
Sunlight and vitamin D	Antacids which contain aluminium
A vegetarian diet	Sugar
Vitamin C – improves calcium absorption	Fluoride and chlorine in drinking water
Whole grains	Too many dairy products
Weight training	Sedentary lifestyle
Zinc	Alcohol

Experiment to find out whether you are better off without natural live yoghurt. Cut it out along with all the other dairy products for a fortnight and see how you feel.
● Refined foods such as white bread, white rice, white pasta and most breakfast cereals, which are not only refined but riddled with sugar.
● Sugar.
● Soya-based ersatz meat substitutes.
● Margarines and golden oils.
● Fried foods. Use only small amounts of extra virgin olive oil or cold-pressed soya oil if you must fry something.
● Coffee, tea and colas – and avoid cigarettes.

Nutritional Support

Calcium

The best source of calcium is not supplements but foods; it is rarely necessary to take calcium supplements. Never take calcium on its own. Instead, change your diet so that you are getting high calcium in foods – preferably not milk products. The ratio of calcium to magnesium is eight to one in milk – far too high. When magnesium isn't absorbed in proper relation to calcium, the calcium does not end up in the bones. It is more likely to lead to inflammatory areas, tendonitis, carpel tunnel syndrome, arthritic spurs and extra calcium deposits around tendons. The doctor will probably call it arthritis or rheumatism or whatever and, because he or she has not been trained in nutrition, will not have the slightest clue that it is a calcium–magnesium imbalance.

Get your calcium from plants: whole grains and vegetables, especially sea vegetables. Calcium is not in the roots but in the structure of a plant – the leaves, the stems and the stalks – and it is not at all difficult to get 600 to 800 milligrams of calcium a day from plant sources. Research suggests that the megadoses of calcium supplements which many women take may actually decrease bone strength and in animal studies have been shown to induce internal bleeding.

Vegetarians and those on a good, moderate-protein diet need only 500 to 600 milligrams of calcium a day. Eating whole-some unprocessed foods makes this easy – especially if you include sea plants in your menus. Calcium is found in good quantities in whole grains such as rye, wheat, millet, brown rice and quinoa as well as pulses and legumes. These foods are also rich in magnesium. Spinach also contains high levels of calcium, but it is high in oxalic acid too, which decreases calcium absorption. Therefore it should not be relied on as a calcium source. If you decide to take some form of calcium supplement, choose a chelated calcium or calcium citrate rather than the usual calcium carbonate or one of the other cheap versions which are not well absorbed. Also consider using betaine hydrochloride.

Remember that once calcium is out of the stomach and in the bloodstream, you have to get it into your bones. This is where exercise comes in, and progesterone (or, in a man's case, testosterone). Exercise will be dealt with in Step Nine. Here is a list of common foods and the amount of calcium each contains:

Calcium Content of Food and Drink

Vegetables	Calcium per cupful (cooked)
Beet greens	165 mg
Broccoli	175 mg
Chinese leaves	125 mg
Kale	180 mg
Mustard greens	100 mg
Pak choi	200 mg
Parsley	122 mg
Turnip greens	250 mg
Wild greens	350 mg

Pulses and legumes	Calcium per cupful (cooked)
Black beans	135 mg
Chickpeas	150 mg
Pinto beans	130 mg
Soya beans	130 mg

Sea vegetables	Calcium per cupful (cooked)
Agar agar (dry flakes)	400 mg
Dulse	570 mg
Hiziki	300 mg
Kelp (kombu)	520 mg
Wakame	520 mg

Mineral water	Calcium per litre
Contrexeville	450 mg
Perrier	140 mg
San Pellegrine	200 mg

Nuts	Calcium per cup
Almonds	300 mg
Brazil nuts	260 mg
Hazelnuts	282 mg

Soya products	Calcium in 112 grams (4 oz)
Tempeh	170 mg
Tofu precipitated with calcium salts	300 mg
Tofu soya-bean curd	100 mg

Other foods	Calcium
Blackstrap molasses	140 mg per tablespoon
Spirulina	30 mg
Tahini	120 mg per 14 grams ($1/2$oz)

In Comparison

Dairy products	Calcium
Cheese	200 mg per 28 grams (1 oz)
Low-fat cheese	150 mg per cup
Milk	300 mg per cup
Non-fat yoghurt	295 mg per cup
Skimmed milk	285 mg per cup

Hydrochloric Acid

One of the major factors in ensuring you get enough calcium is adequate hydrochloric acid in the stomach. In order to get calcium from the stomach into the bloodstream, two things are required: plenty of hydrochloric acid and sufficent B vitamins. A lack of either will stop the absorption of calcium, allowing it to pass through and out of the body, doing nothing for the bones. As they get older many women do not produce enough hydrochloric acid in their stomachs to absorb calcium. An important question to ask yourself is, 'Are there foods I used to be able to eat but now can't?' If there is even the slightest indication that this applies to you, a supplement of hydrochloric acid, usually in the form of betaine hydrochloride, can be useful. A lot of indigestion comes not (as the television ads would have us believe) from 'over-acidity', but rather from a lack of hydrochloric acid. Supplementing main meals with hydrochloric acid also improves the digestion of proteins and can help prevent indigestion and food sensitivities caused by protein foods not being broken down properly in the stomach.

Magnesium

Sixty per cent of the body's magnesium is contained within the bones. Although it makes up only 0.1 per cent of bone (compared with calcium's 20 per cent), magnesium is vital to good bone formation, as it both increases the absorption of calcium from the foods we eat and enhances its role in mineralising bones. In one study that compared magnesium levels in the bones of women with osteoporosis with those of women without it, researchers found that low levels of magnesium are common in women whose bone density and strength has been lost. Magnesium is an element in which women tend to become progressively deficient as they get older, especially if they have been living on a diet of processed foods, because the commercial processing of grains and other foods depletes them of magnesium. Dairy products and muscle meat are low in magnesium and chemical fertilisers leach it from the soil. Sugar and alcohol consumption lead to magnesium loss via the urine. Drinking colas that are high in phosphate greatly decreases magnesium levels. There is practically nothing that happens in your body that isn't related in one way or another to your levels of magnesium. Foods high in magnesium include black-eyed peas, curry, almonds, whole grains and pulses, eggs, liver and green vegetables.

Vitamin D

This vitamin is necessary for the transportation of calcium and phosphorus into bone tissue. It also helps to prevent too much calcium being lost via the urine. The best sources of vitamin D are natural sunlight and natural fish oils.

Zinc

This mineral is also essential for the formation of new bone and, like magnesium, it is processed out of our foods. Zinc deficiencies have now become so widespread that supplementing the diet with zinc appears to be important for many people. Zinc levels tend to be low in women with osteoporosis and in women who take calcium supplements.

Vitamin C

Another important player in the bone-formation game, Vitamin C levels decline as women age. They are also drastically reduced by exposure to pollutants in the air including cigarette smoke. A couple of extra grams of vitamin C each day can protect bones as well as enhance overall health and good looks.

Silicon

An important trace element for the formation of skin, bone, cartilage, hair and nails, silicon also helps to protect the body from some of the damage caused by aluminium in the system. Silicon is an unusual element. It is the second most widespread element in nature, after oxygen. Silica, the organic form of silicon, is enormously hard and has the ability to bind into tissues other minerals which are needed there. Silica is readily available in unprocessed vegetables, but hard to come by when eating processed foods or foods grown chemically. This is why supplements of silica can be useful. It can also be taken in the form of horsetail tea (this plant has the highest content of the trace element – see page 140) and can do wonders for the condition of nails, hair and skin.

Boron

Only recently has boron, another trace element, been thought to be important as a nutrient. The presence of boron reduces calcium loss and increases the level of some of the oestrogens in the body. Boron also affects hormone levels in women and appears to help to normalise them. It has been shown to improve the metabolism of calcium, phosphorous and magnesium, and to aid the manufacture of vitamin D by the body. Alfalfa and kelp are good sources of boron, as are some of the other seaweed foods.

Vitamin B$_6$

Working together with magnesium, this member of the B complex vitamins supports the production of progesterone and encourages the formation of new collagen. A number of studies indicate that women with osteoporosis have low levels of this vitamin.

Typical Supplementation for Osteoporosis

Magnesium 300–600 mg a day in divided doses as magnesium citrate or chelated magnesium
Vitamin D 350–400 iu a day
Zinc 15–20 mg a day as zinc citrate or picolinate
Vitamin C 2000–4000 mg a day in divided doses
Silica As horsetail tea
Boron 2–8 mg a day
Vitamin B$_6$ 50 mg a day before bed

Progesterone

Progesterone plays a significant role in creating good, strong bones. When it is present in optimal quantities it spurs the osteoblasts to make new bone. Some remarkable results have been reported by doctors who in the last twenty years have used progesterone creams. Progesterone has brought relief from pain caused by osteoporosis, stabilised height, reduced the number of fractures, and improved bone density, regardless of age, even in women who already have osteoporosis. The results apply both to women who have used progesterone cream alone and to those who have used small doses of oestrogen as well. Apply the cream daily, using one jar a month, initially for three months. Later half the amount per month may suffice, depending on bone density tests.

When height has been lost as a result of crush fractures in the vertebrae, the pressure on the nerves is often alleviated by progesterone cream and exercise such as walking in a warm swimming pool with the water up to the chest; the buoyancy of the water takes the weight off the spine. This can help the bones to relocate themselves the micro-millimetre distance it takes to relieve pain.

Because natural progesterone applied in cream form has so many other benefits and virtually no side-effects, it would seem unwise for a woman who has any indication of bone loss or who is concerned about preventing osteoporosis not to use it. The nutrients listed in this section are important for progesterone to be efficiently used by the body. It generally takes about three months to begin to experience the sense of wellbeing which generally accompanies progesterone treatment. If you have been diagnosed as having osteoporosis, it is advisable to have serial vertebral bone density studies done at intervals of six months to a year to monitor progress.

Step Nine
Get Moving

THE next time you get the chance, watch how an animal moves. Look at the rhythmic lope of a wolf, its body almost becoming the motion, or a horse in a field, tossing its mane, pounding its hooves and charging about for sheer pleasure. For many years I wondered why after childhood most of us no longer experience this kind of explosive, rhythmical freedom and energy. Why is it we so often feel only half alive? And why do we as women tend to look upon our bodies as separate from ourselves, something to be criticised, judged, or pushed and shoved into shape, instead of celebrating the body's power and joy of movement the way animals do? For too many of us our primary experience of the body is one of deadness. And since none of us is able to live with deadness for long we are forced to seek artificial stimulus through drugs, or alcohol, compulsive work or sex, just to feel alive again. The trouble is, none of the artificial things that we turn to in an attempt to recover our aliveness ever works for very long. Step Nine asks: where does the real key lie?

Mighty Muscle

The answer to this question may surprise you. It stunned me when I first came upon it because it is so simple. The key to aliveness is to be found within the body itself – in muscle tissue. Muscle is the engine that turns food calories into energy, fuels immune functions, burns fat and creates simple joy in whatever you may be doing. In fact it is the cells of muscle tissue that create the life energy for you to think, to move and to feel. To create a strong body and mind you need to nurture and develop your muscle. The better it gets, the greater your experience of aliveness will be. And this is true no matter what your age or state of physical fitness.

Women often talk about the body as if it were a machine. In reality your body is nothing like a machine. A machine, as you use it, wears out. Your body was designed to move. The more you use it, the stronger it becomes. Lack of exercise together with a high-protein diet full of excess meat, eggs, and dairy products, is not only largely responsible for widespread osteoporosis but many other ailments, from PMS and fibroids to breast cancer. We have become a culture of couch potatoes. The adage 'Use it or lose it' really does apply when it comes to the health and good looks of women in mid-life.

Secrets of Muscle

A woman's body thrives on exercise – especially after the age of thirty-five. This is an evolutionary truth which in the last fifty years we have ignored to our peril. Numerous studies show that most bodily changes associated with age have little to do with years passing. They are instead the result of shifts in our lean body mass to fat ratio – that is, decreased muscle mass and increased fat – which occur as a result of simply not using muscle. There is a widespread belief that as women get older their body metabolism naturally slows down and there-fore it is normal that we grow steadily fatter. Once again, the culprit is not the passing of the years but inactivity. Take heart. It doesn't matter how old you are, you can begin now to enhance your lean body mass by increasing the amount of muscle in your body. In the process you will reverse most of the changes attributed to ageing and rejuvenate your body.

Animal bodies, like ours, are made up of two basic components: lean body mass (LBM), which encompasses muscle tissue, and fat. Lean body mass – that part of each of us which is not fat – is the part which is truly alive. It consists of organs such as the heart, liver, brain, pancreas, bones and skin, as well as muscle tissue. Your LBM is vital. It demands oxygen, uses nutrients from your food, thinks and feels, moves, grows and repairs itself. Wild animals have a high percentage of LBM. That is what gives them their power, their ease of movement, their stamina and their sleek bodies. The rest of the body is fat. The hardest thing for women who have been brainwashed by low-calorie slimming nonsense to understand is that if you struggle with a spreading waistline it is your body's fat stores that are the enemy, not your weight as measured by the scales. Build your lean body mass through regular weight-bearing exercise and slowly but inexorably the excess fat will go – again, regardless of age. Fat tissue is very different from muscle. It does not need oxygen, does not create movement or activity, and cannot repair itself. In fact, body fat is just about as close as you can get to dead flesh within a living system. Dr Vince Quas, an American expert on exercise as a tool for personal transformation and the author of an excellent book *The Lean Body Promise*, says it better than anyone else: 'Your lean body mass is you. Your fat is on you.'

Energy Matters

Women in the West lose on average 3.5 kilos (nearly 8 lb) of muscle and gain 10.5 kilos (23 lb) of fat between the ages of twenty and forty. Such a major shift in the ratio of lean body mass to fat in a woman's body does much to undermine the functioning of the immune system and the hormonal system. Aerobic exercise, which we have been encouraged to practise, offers little to protect muscle mass from shrinking. For that you need resistance exercise such as weight-training. In fact the latest research shows that in stressing aerobic exercise above all other kinds for cardiac fitness and overall wellbeing we have been getting the balance wrong for years.

Break your arm and it will shed half its muscle and a third of its bone mass within a few weeks, simply because you have stopped using it. When the cast is taken off it will have shrunk by as much as half its size. If you are forced for any reason to stay in bed for a few months, the loss of minerals from your bones and the ageing of your muscle tissue can speed up by ten years. But the up side is great: your body responds amazingly to exercise – even to a little of it. Begin making demands upon your muscles by doing both aerobic and weight-bearing exercise – start nice and easy, especially if you are not used to exercise. From the very first hour you begin, not only will your muscles grow stronger and smoother, your bone tissue will become denser. But stop exercising again and your energy levels will drop, your muscle mass will shrink, your firm body will begin to go flabby, and you will lose your overall sense of wellbeing.

As yet few women – and few doctors and scientists – realise that how your body performs, chemically as well as physiologically, and how resistant you are to ageing and degenerative disease are determined not by how much or how little you weigh but by the ratio of LBM to fat in your body. A high LBM means high energy. It also means you can eat as much as you like of good, wholesome foods without gaining weight – no matter what your age. And what is even more interesting is that recent research has made it clear that it is a good LBM to fat ratio which heightens immunity and strengthens the body against deterioration of any kind.

Wages of Fear

For a few women, exercise is such a normal part of their lives that they exercise regularly without thinking. It makes them feel good, so they run, swim, play tennis, do yoga, row or attend dance or aerobic classes. For most of us, however, heavier exercise is something that can seem rather daunting, especially if we haven't done any for thirty years. From our earliest introduction to physical activity in schools our perception of exercise is coloured by the confusion that exists between sports skills and fitness. Being skilful at a particular sport does not necessarily have much to do with being fit.

Many women who discovered in school that they were not natural athletes are still put off the idea of taking up some form of regular activity because they feel they lack physical prowess, that they will simply be 'no good at it'. This is completely irrelevant. What matters is simply that you use your body by setting it in motion and letting it experience the kind of movement for which it was made. It can be useful to look at whatever your own unconscious assumptions may be regarding exercise so you can clear away any cobwebs. Exploring the possibilities of what exercise can do to change you for the better – your health and good looks as well as your view of yourself – is a life-expanding experience. It can be one of the most exciting journeys a woman can take at any time but especially in the middle of her life. And this is particularly true if, like me, your natural tendency is to curl up into a ball and flop on to the sofa.

Vital Statistics

Dr Walter Bortz of the Department of Medicine at the Palo Alto Medical Clinic in California published a fascinating paper in which he reviewed more than a hundred studies showing that the sedentary lifestyle which has developed in the past fifty years in the West causes bodily damage. Disuse through inactivity increases levels of cholesterol and reduces vital capacity – your ability to take up and use oxygen. When your body doesn't use oxygen well, your brain and muscles, organs and skin suffer damaging oxygen deprivation and you feel chronically low in energy. Bortz found that the average sedentary forty-five-year old has lost half of the ability to take up and use oxygen. With that loss comes all sorts of degenerative changes to the body that even most doctors still think are a part of normal ageing. But what is so wonderful is that when a sedentary person starts doing regular weight-bearing exercise plus a little aerobic activity for a year, it can restore their ability to take up and use oxygen to that of a twenty-five-year-old. The benefits of restoring vital capacity are superior to any drug or medical treatment in existence. This is particularly true for women in mid-life and beyond. As one of the world's foremost authorities on exercise, nutrition and good health, Dr Michael Colgan, says: 'There is no longer any doubt: exercise can save your life, while couch potatoism creates an existence that is nasty, sick and short . . . Exercise directly prevents disease.'

Your LBM is always shifting. Being inactive makes it shrink. So does going on and off slimming diets. Crash dieting causes you to shed muscle tissue. Yet when lost weight is regained it is regained in fat, forever decreasing the weight of your LBM. This is why the more you diet the flabbier your body becomes. And because crash dieting shrinks LBM, it also shrinks your metabolism. It becomes harder and harder to stay thin, until finally you need to starve yourself (and often ruin your health) to keep the scales right. It is little wonder that when your muscle tissue is as good as it is in a wild animal or healthy child, your own brand of radiance shines through. What I didn't know until recently, however, is that the more you strengthen your LBM, the easier it is to get rid of psychological hang-ups, fears, and all those other niggling things that hold you back, and the more you begin to live your own truth, quite simply and joyously. When it comes to using exercise as a bridge to freedom in mid-life – a way of enhancing your health, regenerating and rejuvenating your body and freeing you from the ravages of twentieth-century women's problems – it's muscle you need to work with. To do so brings about a fascinating metamorphosis and a highly individual one. It will not change you in any intrinsic way, nor will it turn you into someone else's idea of who you should be or what you should look like. It will only help to make you more – in essence – who you are. Working week after week with the right kind of exercise even a body which may have been distorted over the years through stress, poor eating, and lack of movement, will metamorphose into the true form hidden within it. That is where resistance exercise comes in and the best form of resistance exercise is weight training.

Catalogue of Rewards

Working with weights does not mean that you will end up with a hard 'killer' body, or look like the people on the front of weight-lifting magazines. Quite the contrary. Exercise to build muscle – using light weights and many repetitions – is the most effective way of enhancing LBM. It chisels and defines arms, legs, torso, hips and bottom, even if they have been neglected for many years and have lost their natural tone and shape. So good is this kind of body building at improving LBM that until recently no one considered that it might be an excellent form of protecting against degenerative illnesses such as coronary heart disease as well. There was a time when aerobic exercise was considered king for health, fitness and longevity. Now, thanks to new research into the effects of weight training at prestigious centres such as McMasters University in Ontario, we know that aerobic exercise combined with weight training is the very best you can get for health, fitness and longevity as well as good looks, stamina and energy. As a result the much respected American College of Sports Medicine have recently revised their long-standing assertion that aerobic exercise holds the key. Their new programme advises a minimum of two sessions of weight training a week using ten different exercises to enhance the large muscles of the chest, back and legs as well as three sessions of aerobic exercise. I think three sessions a week are needed, each of between thirty minutes to one hour, in which you combine resistance movement with some aerobic activity to warm up and cool down. There you get the best of both worlds. Be sure too to walk as much as you can in the open air.

The right exercise also helps to prevent degenerative diseases such as cancer and heart disease. An eight-year study which followed more than ten thousand men and three thousand women was reported in the *Journal of the American Medical Association* not long ago. It looked at the long-term effects of physical fitness and found that sedentary women – women who are not fit and therefore have a low LBM to fat ratio – have a 460 per cent higher mortality rate than those who take exercise more regularly. Men in the low fitness category had a 340 per cent higher rate.

Exercise Brings Benefits	Disuse Brings Trouble
Builds strong bones.	Renders bones porous and fragile.
Increases life-expectancy, on average by seven years.	Precipitates deterioration of arteries.
Clears anxiety and depression.	Lowers noradrenaline levels and makes you more subject to depression.
Enhances mental clarity.	Induces fuzzy-mindedness.
Enhances immune functions and lowers cancer rates in women.	Encourages aches and pains to develop and suppresses immune function.
Encourages more restful sleep and greater relaxation.	Fosters emotional instability.
Improves both mental and physical flexibility.	Makes ligaments and tendons lose strength and flexibility so you are more easily injured.
Increases mental and physical energy.	Causes muscle and brain cells to lose the capacity for maintaining energy.
Increases insulin sensitivity, helps to maintain energy levels and protect against diabetes.	Undermines energy and encourages blood sugar disturbances and disorders in glucose metabolism.
Improves the elimination of wastes.	Contributes to the development of constipation, haemorrhoids and varicose veins, and can lead to disturbances in bowel function.
Alleviates symptoms of PMS.	Exacerbates symptoms of PMS.
Lowers cholesterol.	Increases levels of cholesterol.
Encourages good lean body mass to fat ratio.	Encourages flabbiness and the laying down of fat stores in the body.
Normalises blood pressure.	Fosters rising blood pressure as the years pass.
Keeps sex hormones at optimum levels.	Causes sex hormones to decline affecting skin, psyche and libido.

Caterpillars into Butterflies

I have always been fascinated by the idea of transformation. You know the kind of thing: frogs into princes, Cinderella into belle of the ball. Most people believe that in real life transformation is not possible. They have never learned to work with muscle. Quite apart from all the mind-boggling new research into how the right kind of exercise can rejuvenate your body, I have discovered for myself that exercise is a great deal more than something you do to counteract ageing or protect yourself from heart disease. It can be used to fan the flames of creativity and help make you more true to yourself. Not only is such transformation possible, it is virtually guaranteed – provided you are patient and provided you are willing to work hard.

Recently I decided to explore just what kind of transformation was possible by working intensively with muscle. I knew that skilful weight training (not the slap-about kind you see carried out in most gyms) is the fastest and most efficient way to do this. So I searched out someone who could work intensively with me as a trainer to shift the LBM to fat ratio in my own body. I found a Welsh champion weight lifter, Rhodri Thomas, who said he would take me on. When we began to work together I was scared to death that after the first two hours I would collapse in a heap. After all, I am no athlete. We trained six days a week. Every day we would work with weights backed up by aerobic exercise such as running, swimming and cycling interspersed with other activities like squash and tennis – just for relaxation. I found to my amazement that I did not collapse. Instead I watched as all sorts of deep changes began to take place. Muscles I didn't know existed slowly and quietly began to surface through my flesh. I discovered that feelings, thoughts and past experience are indeed held within the body. All sorts of old memories, emotions, and fears seemed in some mysterious way to be locked in my muscles. When you work muscle intensively, such things sometimes rise to the surface to be cleared away, much as the body is cleared of physical toxins during a detox programme. Frequently I found myself pushed to my absolute limits. Then the gym floor would be covered equally with my sweat and my tears.

I have discovered that working with muscle in this way transforms the body externally by changing LBM to fat ratio and reshaping the body, which brings all sorts of wonderful rewards, including more energy, freedom from aches and pains, a lean, firm body and better hormonal balance. Even more wonderfully, it creates an internal transformation, developing from within a slow but steadily growing sense of self-confidence, clarity and independence. For many – myself included – this is a deep change virtually impossible to achieve in any other way. So now when I think back to all those fairy tales about transformation, about frogs and princes, for the first time in my life I feel I am beginning to understand them and to understand what real transformation is about. It is not all glitzy, like it is in the movies. It is slow and inexorable. Yet it brings in its wake gifts far beyond our wildest dreams. Now I wonder, would Cinderella have been prepared for union with her Prince Charming had she not for many years before strengthened her body and purified her spirit through hard work?

Second Coming

Exactly what kind of exercise is the right kind? This is an important question to answer because so much of what has become fashionable – fancy clothing and tossing weights around in a gym – is the wrong kind. Walking or running along roads filled with air pollution and subjecting your body to the stress this brings can also do more harm than good. Aware of the benefits of exercise, most people who exercise regularly do aerobic movement: swimming, cycling, running or walking. There is much to be said for this kind of exercise. It improves the functioning of the heart, lowers cholesterol, and shifts brain chemistry so that you produce natural opiates which make you feel good. It also increases noradrenaline, a brain chemical which improves your self-image and confidence so that you feel even better about yourself and about your life. Aerobic exercise can also enhance your body's ability to burn fat not only while you are working out but for many hours afterwards as well. This makes aerobic exercise an important part of any good exercise programme. So get out and walk briskly as often as you can. But aerobic exercise doesn't go far enough. It does not offer the body enough weight resistance to maintain muscle mass.

One interesting study compared the LBM to fat ratio in three groups of women: non-exercisers, aerobic exercisers, and weight trainers. Researchers found significant differences. In sedentary women, 21.8 per cent of their body weight was fat. Among the aerobic exercisers 16.2 per cent was fat, while among resistance trainers only 14.7 per cent of their body weight was fat. Exercise physiologists have come to realise that although aerobic exercise has a place as part of an exercise programme it does not maintain bones and muscle the way resistance exercise does. The bottom line is that we need both, although resistance exercise is the more important of the two. In an official statement, a member of the advisory board of The American College For Sports Medicine – who in the past promoted aerobic exercise as the best form for overall health and fitness – advised: 'Done correctly, weight training is the most efficient, effective, and safest form of exercise there is, and it won't be long before people realise it.'

Where to Begin

First, get an OK from your doctor to make sure that there is no reason you should not start on a simple graded programme of exercise. Then go easy. If you start small and work up you will win. If you start big you may not only wear out your body but also lose your taste for movement; all your effort will have become counter-productive, since you will end up hating exercise and getting nowhere. For exercise to work, it has to become an ordinary part of your daily life. It needs to be done regularly at least three times a week. Begin with just fifteen minutes in the morning when you get up, or at any other time of the day that is convenient. The great news is that right from that very first session your body will begin to rejuvenate itself. Exercise routines progress well when you work out at the same time each day. Try to do this if you can. Your body will get used to the routine and love it. When it comes to resistance training you don't need to own a lot of fancy equipment. Nor do you need to join a gym. A couple of dumbbells will do. Later on if you catch the exercise bug you might like to have a barbell as well. Dumbbells and barbells are what are known as free weights, as opposed to the kind of gym equipment you find in a multitude of sizes and shapes and glitzy finishes these days. Beginners are often dazzled by the high-tech stuff in gyms but, as any serious weight trainer will tell you, for most exercises free weights are far better. They are also far simpler, because you can tuck them quickly under the bed when they are not in use and you can use them any time you want without having to dress up in special clothes and go to the gym.

You will need a pair of dumbbells (one for each hand). Choose the kind that have six removable weights on each so you can add and then take off weights as needed for each exercise. When you are not using the dumbbells, stash them away out of sight. Your body and their weight against gravity offer all the resistance you need to work muscles deeply. The machines you find in gyms are designed to mimic the effects of free weight exercises, but – with a couple of minor exceptions – no matter how flash they look, they are not as good as simple free weights, because they restrict your range of movement. Once you get into weight training and gain a bit of confidence with it, you might find it fun to work out in the gym using these machines occasionally. But free weights should form the basis of any good weight-training routine, whether you are a complete beginner – as I was – or a professional weight lifter.

There are three things you want to accomplish on your exercise programme. First, you want to maintain and to improve your heart and lung fitness. For this you will use weights plus some form of aerobic activity for warming up and cooling down. Second, you want to maintain and increase your muscle mass. Finally, you want to maintain and improve your flexibility. For this you need to incorporate some kind of slow stretching after exercise.

Warm Up

It is important at the beginning of any exercise session that you spend a few minutes doing an aerobic activity. You must never pick up a weight when your muscles are cold. This can be running on the spot, slow, steady jumping jacks, using a rowing machine (my favourite) or bouncing on a rebounder. To begin with, your total exercise session may last only fifteen to twenty minutes, in which case you will want to devote five minutes at the beginning to the aerobic warm-up. Later on it can be longer. I generally row on the rowing machine for about ten minutes at a slow, steady pace to get my heart and lungs moving and warm up before beginning my weights. As the length of your exercise session grows week by week, until it is ideally forty-five minutes to an hour at a time, so will the time you spend on your aerobic activities at the beginning and end of the session and perhaps in the middle too.

Stretch Out

After this initial warm-up period, which should last long enough for you to feel fully warmed up, you should spend five to ten minutes stretching. Stretch slowly and smoothly towards the ceiling, towards your toes, to the side; never jerk when stretching. Breathe deeply. Stretching before a workout and after a warm-up is done to allow major muscle groups along with associated tendons and ligaments to be gently stretched, reducing the possibility of injury. Now you are ready for your muscle work.

Work It Out

To work with weights properly you need to split your sessions into different body parts and work one or two body parts per session, leaving at least forty-eight hours between that session and the next time you work that body part. The muscle and bone strengthening that comes with resistance training does not take place while you are using the weights. In fact, working out stresses the muscles and bones, causing tiny breakdowns in the cells to occur. It is during the rest that comes after a workout that new muscle and bone are built. If you reach the stage where you are using quite heavy weights and training five times a week, it is important to work out each body part only once a week, because it can take forty-eight hours for the breakdown process to take place and between forty-eight and seventy-two hours to build new strong tissue to replace it. Ignorant of these facts, many gung-ho body builders and weight trainers over-train their muscles, undermining their immune system as a result while getting nowhere near the benefits in terms of strengthening LBM that they should. Exercising a particular muscle group every five to eight days is ideal for optimum progress.

Stand in any gym and watch weight trainers do their stuff. It can be highly instructive, showing you how not to work with weights. Ninety per cent of the men and women who use weights let their bodies swing all over the place; when they are doing an exercise such as a dumbbell curl they let the weight just fall back after each movement instead of being in control. When you work out, be sure to keep your body absolutely centred with each movement, only using the particular muscle group that is supposed to be working, and emphasise the return movement where you are returning the weight to its original position. Resist the movement all the way back. It is the stress placed on your muscles of lengthening again when they are under resistance load that brings about most of the gains in strength and LBM you are after. Also make sure that you drink lots of water while you are working out.

The Cool Down

It is important to spend a few minutes at the end of a weights session doing some kind of aerobic activity to cool down. How long depends on the length of your weights session. You can go through the same kind of activity you used at the beginning of your session or even take a brisk walk, but to ensure you stay warm, add an extra sweater. After a workout your body cools down fast and you don't want to become chilled.

Stretch Out Again

Then do some more stretching for a couple of minutes. You will find that your body stretches more easily now, because your muscles are full of blood and energised. Go slowly and enjoy the feeling. It can be wonderful.

Beginner's Programme

You will find pictures of the movements below illustrated in any standard book on weight training. Alternatively, ask a fitness instructor to demonstrate them for you. All the exercises are classic weight-training movements. They are simple and straightforward. They require nothing more than a couple of dumbbells, the kind that have six weights on each which can be unscrewed and changed to give you the right weight for a particular exercise. Start with the lightest weights. You will be able to tell for yourself if something feels right. Never strain. As your body becomes accustomed to the lighter weight you can add a bit more. The object of the exercise is not to use heavy weights, but to create enough resistance for your muscles to work against. Each exercise is done smoothly and with complete control, both on the contraction of the muscle group and on the relaxation. While one muscle group is working the rest of the body remains still and centred.

Start off by doing only three training sessions a week with

one set per exercise. A set is the same exercise repeated a certain number of times. 2 x 10 would mean ten repetitions of the movement, rest for two to three minutes, then ten more repetitions of the movement. 3 x 10 means the ten repetitions are done three times, again with two minutes' rest between each set. Work up to a longer workout by adding more exercises for each muscle group you are working with and doing one warm-up set of easy repetitions (ten to fifteen) followed by a heavier set using a little more weight (five to ten repetitions). Begin with very light weights, just enough for you to feel that your muscles are being worked as you near the end of your repetitions. When you are ready to add your second set, add a little more weight until, at the end of your repetitions, your muscles feel tired.

Session One: Shoulders and Arms

Dumbbell press 2 x 10
Side lateral raise 2 x 10
Single arm tricep extension 2 x 10
Tricep kickback 2 x 10
Dumbbell curl 2 x 10
Concentration curl 2 x 10

Session Two: Chest and Back

Dumbbell bench press 2 x 10
Dumbbell flies 2 x 10
Single arm rowing 2 x 10
Dumbbell shrug 2 x 10
Floor hyperextensions 2 x 10

Session Three: Legs and Abdominal Muscles

Dumbbell squat 2 x 10
Dumbbell lunge 2 x 10
Calf raise 2 x 10
Abdominal crunch 2 x 10–15
Reverse crunch 2 x 10–15

Advanced Workout

Once you have acquired a taste for weights and are training three times a week, you can begin doing longer sessions – up to forty-five minutes to one hour. You might also like to do more sessions per week moving up from three to five. Then you would divide your body-part work like this:

Session One: Shoulders

Dumbbell press 1 x 12, 2 x 8
Side lateral raise 1 x 12, 2 x 8
Bent lateral raise 1 x 12, 2 x 8
Front lateral raise 2 x 10

Session Two: Back

Dumbbell dead lift 1 x 12, 3 x 8–10
Single arm rowing 3 x 10
Floor hypers 3 x 10–12
Dumbbell shrugs 3 x 10

Session Three: Chest

Dumbbell bench press 1 x 12, 3 x 8–10
Dumbbell pullover 1 x 12, 2 x 8–10
Dumbbell flies 3 x 10

Session Four: Arms

Single arm tricep extension 1 x 12, 3 x 8
Tricep extension 3 x 8–10
Dumbbell curl 1 x 12, 3 x 8
Concentration curl 3 x 8–10

Session Five: Legs and Abdominals

Dumbbell squat 1 x 12, 3 x 8
Dumbbell lunge 3 x 10
Dumbbell step up 3 x 12
Stiff leg dead lift 3 x 10
Calf raise 3 x 12

Abdominal crunch 3 x 15–20
Side crunch 3 x 15–20
Reverse crunch 3 x 15–20

The Result

Each woman is in reality two women: an outer woman who can come in many forms – conventionally attractive, plain, sexy, dynamic, withdrawn, aggressive, apparently assured or terribly uncertain about herself – and her inner counterpart, an individual self that is utterly unique. Each woman has a stable centre of strength and growth. Each inner woman sees the world in her own way, has her own brand of creativity, her own needs and desires, and is a law unto herself. The inner self holds the power to create, change, build, nurture and transform. The outer woman is the vehicle for what the self creates. When her inner self is allowed free expression, a woman is truly beautiful, for she is fully alive. Her body is strong, her skin is clear and healthy, and her movements, speech and actions radiate a charismatic vitality that is unmistakably real, an outward expression of who she truly is. Many of the secrets of calling forth this kind of aliveness are to be found within the body itself. They are secrets best learned by working with muscle. Once you get the hang of it, working with weights is like meditation – one of the most mind-stilling activities in the world. Meanwhile, as your LBM begins to develop, you will find that your muscles and whole body have come alive. When you work out, your muscles will begin to glow. After a few months your body will begin to feel the way it did when you were a child – radiant with life and spirit.

Step Ten
Trust Yourself

In the past half century a woman's place as defined by society has undergone drastic shifts and revisions, many of which have offered us greater freedom of choice. Women have demanded, and to some degree achieved, equal opportunities with men in the work place. We have refused to spend all of our lives in supportive roles. We have sought out new ways of relating to our families, work colleagues and friends – as well as to ourselves. We have also gone a long way towards eroding long-standing assumptions about women: the idea that we are too emotional, too unfocused, too fickle to accomplish anything significant. We have proved that women have good minds and are capable of high achievement academically, in business, and in the arts. Yet being a woman in today's world demands that we be willing to live the life of a juggler. Each of us has become involved in a never-ending task of trying to keep the balls of our life's roles in the air – professional woman, mother, worker, lover, wife, achiever – while we get through each day, week and year. In the last step to a natural menopause we look at how a woman can begin to discover the truth of her own personality, and the new life that lies beyond menopause.

Daughters of the Father

Many women have chosen to walk away from the limited, self-sacrificing lives they watched their mothers lead, lives which too often produced grief and bitterness as the menopause years approached. Instead of following in the footsteps of the traditional female, whose primary role was concerned with nurturing, they have looked towards the male world for their mentors and role models, to find ways of giving credence to their need for a sense of purpose, to their ambition and intellect, and to find direction and a definition of success. Other women have simultaneously tried to live out the male ambition inherited from the world of their fathers and to redefine their mothering role, in the hope that they will be successful in the world yet still be able to raise their children and fulfil their sexual and emotional needs. Still others have chosen to dedicate themselves primarily to nurturing the ambitions of lovers or husbands and the development of their children so long as they remain within the family.

These are only a few of the possible choices now open to women in a world where shifting economic, social and personal values have undermined the established social order and made choice possible. Whatever path we choose, each of us searches for meaning and longs for freedom – whenever we have time to think about it between child-rearing, paying the bills, and trying to look as if we have just walked off the cover of *Vogue*. So great are the demands on women now – many of them self-imposed – that we are in danger of losing track of ourselves and burning out. Just as our mothers and their mothers before them embraced the expectations of their culture – that fulfilment would come through being a good wife, a good mother or a good servant – women have now taken on another cultural stereotype. We have learned to do things logically. We have thrown ourselves headlong into the male world and many of us have 'made it' within that world's terms. Yet, in the wake of our success, we often find ourselves pursued by a confusing sense of barrenness and despair that further achievement in the world, new love affairs, or the prospect of a face-lift can do nothing to cure.

Dark Goddess

The fear of menopause and the fear of the crone, so widespread in our society, are nothing more than a reflection of a fear of death itself. In our modern world we have forgotten the great cycle of birth, flowering, death and regeneration. Our patriarchal culture views events as linear, not cyclical. In linear time the end is not connected with the beginning, they are opposites, the one to be celebrated the other to be resisted at all costs until the bitter end. It is no wonder that our society wants to blank out menopause and reject the older woman. Our cultural conditioning has taught us to undervalue the wild feminine within us, that part which is instinctual, irrational, non-moral and full of passion. The society in which we live is so frightened of these things that we ourselves have been taught to fear the feminine within us and judge it harshly. Too often we swallow our anger, even when it is righteous, we put our needs and wants below those of others, and we crush our wild nature. We judge ourselves wrongly and we see ourselves as ugly. Doing so dissipates our power. The most difficult task any woman comes up against is that of accepting the part of herself which she finds most ugly and loathsome. Yet locked within what we most hate and fear lies the greatest potential for freedom.

The wild power of the feminine lives within all of us. She is the part of you that refuses to uphold any relationship that doesn't work. The part of you that has the power to set limits, to shout 'No!' and to say: 'This is what I will do and this is what I won't do' when faced with any sort of abuse or domination. We spend most of our lives trying to avoid crises at any cost. Yet crises are often the only means by which we can make a better life for ourselves. At menopause this part of ourselves demands that we clear out of our lives whatever is left over from our child-bearing years and is no longer appropriate. Ignore its demands and the results can be terrifying. Have you ever noticed how many women go through crisis after crisis at menopause: broken marriages, lost jobs, loss of self-confidence? It seems that this part of your personality will sabotage everything you hold dear, cut through all the feminine images of being 'pleasing', 'submissive', 'gentle', and 'nice', grab you by the throat and pull you under, until you accept that you have a new life to lead.

Call to Adventure

The joy of menopause is the world's best-kept secret. Of course nobody told me this beforehand. It was a secret I had to discover for myself. Like most modern women my head had been filled with the horrors of hot flushes, fainting spells and dry vaginas; with memories of my mother's tears shed over a wrinkle that appeared one day to mar her perfect face; with the prospect of enforced celibacy – after all, no man can feel lust for an old woman, can he? The secret I discovered is that menopause is a call to adventure, a call that can arrive in as many different forms as there are women to hear it. Sometimes it means making a real journey to another place, moving to a new job, or leaving behind a marriage which has outlived its usefulness. For others the journey takes place in the mind.

I was the daughter of a jazz musician. As a child I didn't go to school. I grew up on the road with my father, travelling hundreds of miles a day from one job to the next. Many places where his band played were amusement parks. Amusement parks are wonderful places, full of all sorts of bright lights, games to play, things to do and prizes to be won. However, I remember noticing, at the age of six or seven, how the stark light of dawn revealed every hidden scrap of paper in the park, every surface whose paint had worn. A funfair the morning after is quite a different place from the one it was only hours before. Often a woman's experience of menopause is like this. An amusement park in broad daylight can be terrifying to someone who wants to go on, entranced by the illusory games it offered a few hours before. But to others who have grown tired of the games, it offers new textures and colours – a far richer and truer experience of reality than any number of neon lights and whirling wheels could ever hope to mimic. 'The party's over,' the song says, 'the candle flickers and dims . . . Now you must wake up.' This is the challenge of the menopausal woman. In this challenge lies a choice: try to run back into the world of the funfair, or to step forward towards the clear light of dawn. Take a look at the reality around you and ask the question: 'Where do I go from here?'

Tell the Truth

A good place to start is by telling the truth. This may sound trivial or even beside the point. Yet being able to *be* whomever you are, *say* whatever you think and *feel* without guilt, recrimination or justification whatever you feel breaks down a lot of barriers. It also brings a sense of freedom that we have as children but lose when we take on the trappings and complexities of adulthood. At the core of each of us sleeps our soul, that part that makes us utterly unique and holds within it our goals, characteristics and potential. The more we are aware of the nature of our soul, of its real intentions, and of what brings us joy, the easier it becomes to live out who we are – to tell our truth. Once truth begins to be told it becomes easier and easier to clear out the old behaviour patterns that were so suited to the child-bearing years but are no longer appropriate. As we are able to identify and lift off these things, we release the most enormous amount of creative energy. Think of how you feel when you are doing something you love. Energy just seems to pour forth. Compare this with the way you feel when you lie, compromise, and do your duty. How would you rather feel? Begin to listen to what I call 'the whispers of the soul' – and then, slowly but surely, start putting what they tell you into practice.

Soul Secrets

Most of us have never learned how to do this. Instead we have been taught *not* to listen to our inner voice. We have been filled with all sorts of stuff by our parents, our educational system, our bosses, our spouses and the media, which teaches us not to trust ourselves but rather to live our lives according to external 'rules'. These rules may be homilies like 'Always think of your children first,' 'Don't do it if your husband doesn't want you to,' 'People will stare at you in the street,' 'Be practical.' Or they can come from advertisements that would have us believe that what we *are* is not good enough and that we need a new car, job, image, body, just to be OK. This continuous bombardment creates a lot of 'static' which obscures the whispers of the soul, making it harder to take notice of what we really value, what we really want, or who we really are.

A good exercise is to write down six rules that you live by. My own are things like: I always do what I think is best for my children, I will not work with people I do not respect, and I try to get rest when I need it. When you have chosen your six rules, take a good look at them. Put a tick by those that have come from other people – school, parents, religion, television, so-called friends. How many are you left with that are really your values? It is these values that you need to discover and explore. It takes a little practice to develop the skill of listening to your inner voice. Strangely, the first whispers you hear may make no sense at all. For instance, for many years I longed for a pair of red shoes, but I never bought them. I suppose it felt selfish and trivial to me when I was earning a living to support four children. But also, red shoes seemed *dangerous* to me – the kind of thing a gypsy might wear to dance on a table – something that had no place in the life of a responsible woman like me.

A Passion for Red Shoes

I didn't know why I wanted a pair of red shoes, but it was something I always longed for. There wasn't a lot of extra money for buying red shoes, but one day when I was about thirty-five, in a moment of rashness I went out and I bought myself a pair. I took them home and felt like I had as a child when I had a new pair of black patent shoes. I wandered around for two days staring at my feet. I adored them. From the moment I put them on some part of my personality that I never knew existed started to raise its head. I won't say that I started dancing on tables but whenever I wore them I found myself having a lot of fun. I began to feel that a passionate, wild, and irresponsible side of me that had never been allowed space was sneaking out and enjoying itself.

What I discovered from that experience goes far beyond the trivial action of buying a pair of red shoes. I discovered that the language of the soul is a language not of sense, rationality or virtue. It is a language of metaphor, of passion and imagination. When you begin to listen to inner whispers about relatively trivial things, your inner voice gets louder. Before long you are hearing the answers to much more important questions and getting more vital information about your health, your goals, your values and your life. I would never have written my first novel, something I was very uncertain about and yet longed to be able to do, had I not bought that pair of shoes.

Four Keys to Your Soul

Ask yourself the questions below one at a time. Then, letting your mind roam free, write down whatever comes to you. You may feel that the answer to one demands reams of words while the answer to another is very short. Explore each question fully before going on to the next. The questions are:

Who am I?
This does not mean your name and where you come from but rather what comes to your mind when the question is asked. How do you see yourself? What are you like?

What do I want?
This should include everything you feel you want or anything you secretly dream of, from the tiniest thing such as 'I want to take up tapestry,' or 'I have always wanted to ride a motorbike' to huge desires you may never have dared to voice: 'I want to go off to Africa to help people dig wells,' 'I want to write a novel,' 'I want to own a chain of restaurants.' It doesn't matter, just write it down.

What do I think is stopping me?
Make a note of any circumstance, person, place, thing, thought or feeling that you feel stands in your way.

Where am I right now in relation to what I want?
To create what you want in your life – from greater self-esteem to your dream home – you need two things. First, you need as clear a vision as possible of what it is you are seeking. Second, you need to be certain of where you are right now in relation to that vision. The greater your desire to achieve a goal and the clearer you can be about where you are in relation to that goal, the easier the achievement of that goal becomes.

These four questions do not have pat answers. The answers you give are going to change as you change, so come back to them periodically and reassess how you feel about them.

Plan Your Way

Go back to the answer to the question 'What do I want?' Start with a desire you believe is within your reach – I would start with the smallest and easiest one – and plan how you are going to achieve it. The more definite a plan you make for yourself, the more likely you are to achieve your goal. A definite plan helps you to take seriously what you are doing. It can also be a source of considerable personal insight. Once you are well on your way to achieving that goal, choose another and make another plan, or choose several related goals and work towards them together. Be as specific as possible about each goal, how you are going to work towards it, exactly why you want to achieve this particular goal, and what you intend to gain from it. Record your progress and any setbacks. This will help you to refine both your goals and your values.

Doing this over and over again will gradually allow you to see that you can make the life you want. Learning to set goals is really helpful. It is much easier to achieve something if you set yourself a goal. Achieving one goal is also the biggest incentive to achieving the next one and the best reinforcement for a sense of personal development and power. But be realistic. Big goals are made up of lots of little ones, so remember to take one step at a time. Not reaching unrealistic goals is likely to set you back rather than take you forward.

Act Your Part

When in doubt, act 'as if'. There is a lot of power in this suggestion. Pretence, which many people look askance at and demean, is often the mother of genuine change. The dilettante, whose main interest in painting comes from a desire to impress at parties, may find one day wandering through the National Gallery that, caught unawares between silly statements about the pictures, he or she has been stung by the bee of real aesthetic experience. Many a genuine passion has begun with such pretence and turned into something life-changing. Pretence – not lying and compromise. By 'pretending' to be as strong, healthy, and self-aware as you would like to be, you both raise your expectations and put yourself in the frame of mind that can help to bring these things about. You can programme your subconscious to change your conscious life for the better. If your first goal is to be fit and full of energy, tell your subconscious that you are indeed fit and full of energy, and it will get on the grapevine and tell your conscious mind that you do, indeed, have an abundance of energy.

Break Through

Do not ignore the question 'What do I think is stopping me?' I am willing to bet that one of the things most people put as an answer is: 'I don't have enough money.' This was one of mine. When I decided to write a novel I decided I was not going to be able to do anything about it because I needed every penny I could earn to bring up my children. I couldn't possibly just stop working so that I could write a novel. At the age of about forty-five I found that, through a lucrative project I had been working on, I had all the money I needed to stop working for a while and write my novel. That sounds great. The reality was terrifying. I discovered that it was not lack of money that had been stopping me at all. It was fear of failure. And breaking through that barrier was much harder than earning the money I thought I needed in the first place. Take another look at what you think is stopping you from achieving your goals and ask yourself if that is really what is holding you back. Re-examine the list you made of rules you live by. Are any of them mixed up with the things you think are stopping you? If so, what can you do about them? Be warned: your goals may be nearer than you think.

Sealing the Self

Do not be tempted to sink yourself into achieving goals in the same way that women spend their lives sinking themselves into achieving what they think is expected of them. This is something different. This is the process of natural menopause, which entails uncovering the real you that has been hidden by the responsibilities of the child-bearing years and discovering the freedom that their passing can bring. One of the differences between the pre-menopausal driving towards goals and the post-menopausal search for freedom is knowing when to stop. Continually set aside enough time to restore yourself. Go into the garden and sit, go for walks by yourself, and take time to listen to music, care for yourself, and take your needs seriously.

A woman's progress through the natural menopause is marked with new insights and understandings of who she is and what she needs. Week by week this becomes clearer as an awareness of her own identity begins to emerge. When you begin to experience the freedom this brings, some conscious decisions need to be made. You might decide, for instance, no longer to put your energy into worrying about what is going to happen next and how you are going to survive, choosing instead to use your new-found freedom as creatively as possible in your life. This usually involves searching to find out what brings you the greatest joy and the greatest sense of meaning, then immersing yourself more and more in it as the days go by. The more you do, the more physical energy is likely to be available to you that has been locked up in worry, frustration and negative feelings towards yourself or others. I think this must be what anthropologist Margaret Mead was talking about when she spoke of 'post-menopausal zest'.

Think of one single thing that you enjoy doing and then promise yourself that you will do it, whether it be dancing, tapestry, taking long walks, doing some sort of public service, or learning about a subject that intrigues you, just for the sake of learning. The more you direct your energy the more there seems to be to direct. Mythologist Joseph Campbell used to urge people: 'Follow your bliss.' By this he did not mean going out of your way to have a good time or chasing rainbows. Far from it. It means finding out what is your particular passion and then pursuing it for its own sake, simply because you enjoy it. For women this may be gardening or going back to university or travelling. The whole point about following your bliss is that doing so leads step by step down a road towards the kind of fulfilment that has nothing to do with striving for success or the approval of society. It is rather like rediscovering the joy of being a child when you could sit for hours happily performing one task.

To Catch a Dream

A few years ago a friend gave me a dreamcatcher – a circular mandala-type of wall hanging that comes out of the Native American tradition. Made from leather thong, chamois, beads and feathers, dreamcatchers consist of a circle inside which is woven a web-like structure; from it are hung long pieces of beaded chamois and feathers. A dreamcatcher is hung above the bed. It is designed to catch your dreams. It is said to eat the bad dreams, while your good dreams get caught by the web and, when the web grows fat enough with them, they spill over it to make their way down the beaded chamois, leather, beads and feathers, intensified the way that water flows faster as it spills over a waterfall. So the good dreams are given back to you in abundance.

I had seen one or two dreamcatchers, found them interesting, and had evidently mentioned this to my friend. She decided to gather together what was necessary and make me one. I was fascinated by the beautiful gift. I hung it above my bed and a few nights later became aware that what I wanted to do most was to make a dreamcatcher of my own. I asked her to show me how to weave the web. It turned out to be very easy and I began to make dreamcatcher after dreamcatcher. To my surprise I rediscovered a sense of joy and excitement in what I was doing that I had not experienced since childhood. This is something I have rarely experienced as a writer. I am a woman who, after I have created something, no longer has any interest in it. I have always tended to feel little satisfaction from anything that I have made. I found that working with dreamcatchers was completely different. I would sit in the middle of my studio surrounded by a total chaos of beads and stones, shells and chamois, small pieces of wood and dried flowers, and spend hours at a time twisting things and building upon the webs to create dreamcatchers of great diversity. I learned from making them that you don't have to know exactly where you are going when you begin a task or take up a challenge. You only need to work from one step to the next and trust your instincts. This is what following your bliss is all about.

New Values

My own experience of a natural menopause has made me clear about what I think and what my values are. I believe:

- That each woman is born unique and gifted.
- That creativity is wild and free and female in nature, even when found in a man.

- That too often a woman's creativity is kept within. Unless she takes action herself it tends to remain imprisoned.
- That every woman has a right to walk her own path and speak with her own voice.
- That all life, art, sexuality, wishes and dreams move in cycles, like the flow and ebb of a woman's hormones.
- That as women we have tended to allow our own imprisonment and treat it as normal.
- That a woman must above all honour her instincts.
- That a woman's wild spirit is best fed when she surrounds herself with things she loves and does the things she likes doing best.

I have come to believe that the journey we are called upon to make at menopause is the most important journey a woman ever makes, first because, given her age and maturity, it is taken with the greatest awareness and, second, because at the end of the child-bearing years she has been released from the need to channel her energy into propagating the species. Now, at last, she is free to use her energy, creativity and intelligence in any way she wants. We have been far too busy giving birth, raising children and nurturing the creativity of others to be able to care for ourselves properly and explore our own potential. The journey of menopause offers the possibility of changing these patterns in our lives once and for all. This is the secret, and the joy, of a natural menopause.

Further Reading

Achterberg, Jeanne, *Woman as Healer*, Shambhala, Massachusetts, USA, 1990.

Brown, Ellen and Lynne Walker, *Breezing Through the Change*, Frog Ltd, Berkeley, CA, USA, 1994.

Campbell, Joseph, *The Hero With a Thousand Faces*, Bollingen Foundation, New York, USA, 1972.

Campbell, Joseph, *Primitive Mythology: The Masks of God*, Arkana, Penguin, New York, USA, 1991.

Coney, Sandra, *The Menopause Industry*, Penguin Books, London, 1991.

Dalton, Dr K., 'The Premenstrual Syndrome', *British Medical Journal*, 1953, 1, 1007.

Downing, Christine, *Women's Mysteries*, The Crossroad Publishing Company, New York, USA, 1992.

Dumble, Lynette, and Renata Klein, 'Hormone Replacement Therapy: Hazards, Risks and Tricks', Proceedings of *Menopause: The Alternative Way: Facts and Fallacies of the Menopause Industry*, 1993, Australian Women's Research Centre, Deakin University, Australia.

George, Demetra, *Mysteries of the Dark Moon*, Harper, San Francisco, USA, 1992.

Grant, Dr Ellen, *Sexual Chemistry: Understanding Our Hormones, The Pill and HRT*, Cedar Original, Mandarin Paperbacks, London, 1994.

Grof, Stanislav, and Christina Grof (eds), *Spiritual Emergency*, Jeremy Tarcher Inc, Los Angeles, USA, 1989.

Grof, Stanislav, and Christina Grof, *The Stormy Search for Self*, Jeremy Tarcher Inc, Los Angeles, USA, 1990.

Lee, John R., MD, *Natural Progesterone*, BLL Publishing, California, USA, 1993.

Lee, John R., MD, *Optimal Health Guidelines*, BLL Publishing, California, USA, 1994.

Northrup, Christiane, *Women's Bodies, Women's Wisdom*, Bantam Books, New York, 1994.

Owen, Lara, *Her Blood is Gold*, HarperSanFrancisco, USA, 1993.

Pearl, W., *Keys to the Inner Universe: The Encyclopedia on Weight Training*, Bill Pearl Enterprises, Phoenix, Oregon, 1982.

Pinkola Estes, Clarissa, *Women Who Run With the Wolves*, Rider, London, 1992.

Reitz, Rosetta, *Menopause: A Positive Approach*, Unwin Paperbacks, London, 1985.

Vines, Gail, *Raging Hormones*, Virago, London, 1993.

Weed, Susan S., *Menopausal Years, The Wise Woman Way*, Ash Tree Publishing, New York, 1992.

Resources

More from Leslie Kenton
Leslie's audio tapes, including *10 Steps to A New You*, as well as her videos, including *Ageless Ageing, Lean Revolution, 10 Day De-Stress Plan* and *Cellulite Revolution*, can be ordered from QED Recording Services Ltd, Lancaster Road, New Barnet, Hertfordshire EN4 8AS. Telephone 0181 441 7722. Fax 0181 441 0777. Email: QED@globalnet.co.uk.

If you would like information about Leslie's personal appearances, forthcoming books, videos, workshops and projects, please visit her website for the latest information: http://www.qed-productions/lesliekenton.htm You can also write to her care of QED at the above address enclosing a stamped, self-addressed A4-size envelope.

Society for Complementary Medicine
31 Weymouth Street, London W1N 3FJ
Telephone 0171 436 0821 Fax 0171 436 1877

Founded in 1989, this charitable trust is dedicated to the development of preventative medicine, immune enhancement and holistic clinical treatment. At the society, practitioners see people by appointment. They offer leading-edge treatment using advanced energy medicine including soft laser therapy, microcurrent therapy, magnetic field therapy and homoeopathy as well as advanced nutritional guidance including brain enhancement. The society cares for people fighting common illnesses as well as those striving for optimum health. It offers special care to those challenged with critical illnesses who are unable to afford treatment. Highly recommended.

Centre for Transpersonal Perspectives
7-11 Kensington High Street, London W8 5NP
Telephone 0171 937 9190

This organisation offers excellent workshops and lectures as well as training in transpersonal psychology and personal growth, many of which are helpful for a woman in the midst of profound personal life changes. Write to them for a list of their activities and dates.

Well Woman's International Network

La Breque, Alderney, Channel Islands GY9 3TJ, UK
Telephone 07000 437225 Fax 07000 329 9946

The Well Woman's International Network (WWIN) is an organisation for women to use as a network resource to make contact and stay in touch with natural health developments that can make a vital difference to enjoying life to the full, regardless of age. They offer information on natural supplements and progesterone products. Patron: Dr John Lee. The Network offers a full range of natural hormone products (including vegan) at discounted prices for its members, postal/Email consultation with specialist doctors, and a quarterly forum/newsletter.

Higher Nature Limited

The Nutrition Centre, Burwash Common, East Sussex, TN19 7LX
Telephone 01435 882 880

This is the company which courageously introduced natural progesterone products to the British market, only to find that within a few months they were forced to restrict their sales to prescription only. Their progesterone and oestrogen products are recognised by the Medicines Control Agency as unlicensed medicines available by doctor's prescription under the 'named patient exemption' of the Medicines Act. They give information to medical doctors on the use of their products, which include:

> Pro-Gest Cream: 50 grams (2 oz) of a three per cent natural progesterone cream, from Mexican yam, in a base of vitamin E and aloe vera.
> Pro-Gest Oil 25 grams (1 oz) of a ten per cent natural progesterone oil in a base of vitamin E. Can be used sub-lingually or applied externally.

In addition, Higher Nature offer a small range of first-rate nutritional products which you can order direct. They are all completely vegetarian, hypo-allergenic, innovative in their formulations and freshly prepared. They also provide excellent nutritional and health consultation, both to the medical profession and health practitioners and to the general public by telephone. Write to them for a list of their products and services.

Phyto Products Ltd
Park Works, Park House, Mansfield Woodhouse, Notts NG19 8EF
Telephone 01623 644 334 Fax 01623 657 232

An excellent company originally set up to supply herbalists with high-quality herbs and plant products. Every plant and herb they sell states the source of origin. All Phyto Products' plants are purchased only from recognisable sources. They offer a full range of tinctures, herbal skin creams, fluid extracts, herbs and the Schoenenberger plant juices, plus Calendula cream and Comfrey cream. All the herbs mentioned in this book are supplied by this company in both tincture form and as the loose dried herb. They do not supply herbs in capsules, but they now produce some herbs in tablet form. Write to them for their price list. They set a minimum order limit of £20 (before VAT) plus carriage.

Specialist Herbal Supplies
Freepost (BR1396), Hove, West Sussex BN3 6BR
Telephone 01273 202 401 Fax 01273 705 120
Email: sales@herbalsupplies.com

This company has been supplying high-quality additive-free herbal aids to health practitioners in the UK and abroad since 1982. They now offer a range of good-quality products for the general public as well, offering single herbs and mixtures as capsules, tinctures or extracts. Write to them for their catalogue.

Bioforce (UK) Ltd
Olympic Business Park, Dundonald, Ayrshire, KA2 9BE
Telephone 01563 851 177 Fax 01563 851 173

Suppliers of herbal extracts, tinctures, homoeopathic remedies and natural self-care products and foods, Bioforce are a Swiss company started by the Swiss expert in natural health, Dr Alfred Vogel. The company always use fresh herbs in preparing their products at the Bioforce factory in Roggwil. They supply over a hundred different herbal and homoeopathic preparations, all of which are very high quality. They can be ordered by post but are often also available in good health-food stores and pharmacies carrying herbal products.

Weleda (UK) Ltd
Heanor Road, Ilkeston, Derbyshire, DE7 8DR
Telephone 0115 944 8200 Fax 0115 944 8210
http//www.weleda.co.uk

Weleda grew out of the work of Rudolf Steiner and have been making medicines and body care products for seventy-five years. Weleda UK grow over four hundred species of plants organically and biodynamically for use in their medicines and body-care range. They produce excellent creams and a delightful skin-care range. Weleda products are available from good health stores and pharmacies. Alternatively, order them direct on 0115 944 8222.

BioCare
The Lakeside Centre, 180 Liffard Lane, Kings Norton, Birmingham, West Midlands B30 3NT
Telephone 0121 433 3727 Fax 0121 433 3879

A science-based manufacturer of innovative nutritional and health-care products, BioCare was founded nearly twenty years ago by practitioners for practitioners. BioCare products are now available to the public by mail order (ring for a catalogue) as well as through suppliers of sophisticated nutritional products such as the Nutri Centre. Their oil-based products, from Vitamin E to linseed oil, are all specially formulated to protect from oxidation by flushing each capsule with nitrogen. In the case of light-sensitive products, BioCare use opaque capsules. They even offer chemical-free vitamins in liquid form which have been specially emulsified or micelized to enhance the absorption to ninety-five per cent. These can be added to juice or water or taken sub-lingually. They are excellent for people with allergies or digestive problems. BioCare produce the very highest-quality nutritional products in Britain.

Xynergy Products
Lower Elstead, Midhurst, West Sussex GU29 0JT
Telephone 01730 813 642

Xynergy specialise in the finest aloe vera products and green nutritional products – such as spirulina and cereal grasses – you can buy. They are available in sophisticated health food stores or can be ordered by post direct from them.

The Nutri Centre
7 Park Crescent, London W1N 3HE
Telephone 0171 436 5122 Fax 0171 436 5171

The Nutri Centre is on the lower ground floor of the Hale Clinic in London and has the finest selection of nutritional products and books on health under one roof in Britain. It can also supply herbs, homoeopathic products, Ayurvedic and biochemic products, flower remedies, essential oils, skin-care and dental products, and has an extensive selection of books, including Leslie Kenton's, all available through a good mail-order service.

The Natural Progesterone Information Service
NPIS, Box 131, Etchingham TN19 7ZN

For information on the multiple uses of progesterone for women's health from puberty to menopause, as well as a list of the books, tapes and videos available on the subject, write to the above address.

Progesterone Body Creams and Oils
Dr John Lee states clearly that natural progesterone oils and creams which contain less than 800 milligrams per 50-gram (2-oz) jar will not supply sufficient progesterone if you are truly deficient. The following American products contain 400–500 mg of progesterone per 25 grams:

Angel Care: Angel Care USA, Atlanta, GA
Bio Balance: Elan Care USA, Scottsdale, ZA
Edenn Cream: SNM, Norcross, GA
E'Pro & Estrol Balance: Sarati International, Pasadena, TX
Equilibrium: Equilibrium Lab, Boca Raton, FL
Fair Lady: Village Market, Fond du Lac, WI
Femarone-17: Wise Essentials, Minneapolis, MN
Feminique: Country Life, Hauppage, NY
Happy PMS: HM Enterprises, Inc, Norcross, GA
Kokoro Balance Cream: Kokoro, LLC, Laguna Niguel, CA
Marpe's Wild Yam: Green Pastures, Flat Rock, NC
NatraGest: Broadmore Labs Inc, Ventura, CA
Natural Balance: South Market Service, Atlanta, GA
Natural Woman: Products of Nature, Ridgefield, CN
OstaDerm: Bezwecken, Beaverton, OR

PhytoGest: Karuna Corp, Novato, CR
Pro-Alto: Health Watchers Sys, Scottsdale, AZ
ProBalance: Springboard, Monterey, CA
Pro-G: TriMedica, Scottsdale, AZ
Progessence: Young Living, Payson, UT
Progonol: Bezwccken, Beaverton, OR
Renewed Balance: America Image Marketing, Nampa, ID
Serenity: Health & Science Nutrition, N Lauderdale, FL

You can purchase Pro-Get by post from:

Woman's International Pharmacy
5708 Manova Drive, Madison, WI, USA
Telephone 001 608 221 7800 Fax 001 608 221 7819

Natural progesterone cream is also available from:

Wellsprings Trading Ltd
PO Box 322, St Peter Port, Guernsey, Channel Islands GY1 3TP

Other Products

Flaxseeds/Linseeds
Linusit Gold linseeds are available from the Nutri Centre (see above). Organic linseeds are also available from Higher Nature (see above). Keep them refrigerated.

Ginseng
A good ginseng comes in the form of Jinlin Ginseng Tea, Jinlin *Panax ginseng* dried slices, ampoules and Jinlin whole root, available from health food stores. You can also buy ginseng tea in bags and in instant granulated sachets which I use regularly. If you have difficulty finding them, contact Alice Chiu, 4 Tring Close, Barkingside, Essex, IG2 7LQ (Telephone 0181 550 9900, Fax 0181 554 3883)

Marigold Swiss Vegetable Bouillon Powder
This instant broth made from vegetables and sea salt comes in regular, low-salt, vegan and organic varieties. It is available from health food stores, or direct from Marigold Foods, 102 Camley Street, London, NW1 0PF (Telephone 0171 388 4515, Fax 0171 388 4516)

Organic Foods
The Soil Association publishes a regularly updated *National Directory of Farm Shops and Box Schemes* which costs £3 (including postage) from The Organic Food and Farming Centre, 86 Colston Street, Bristol, BS1 5BB. Excellent organic beef, lamb, port, bacon, ham, chicken, and sausage can be ordered from Longwood Farm Organic Meats, Tudenham St Mary, Bury St Edmunds, Suffolk, IP28 6TB. (Telephone 01638 717 120)

Organics Direct
This company offers a nationwide home delivery service of fresh vegetables and fruits, delicious breads, juices, sprouts, fresh soups, ready-made meals, snacks and baby foods. They also sell the state-of-the-art 2001 Champion Juicer and the 2002 Health Smart Juice Extractor for beginners. They even sell organic wines – all shipped to you within twenty-four hours. Telephone 0171 729 2828, or visit their website on www.organicsdirect.com. You can also order online.

Pure Mail Order
They supply organic foods and natural remedies as well as macrobiotic foods, mail order. They offer herb teas, organic grains, whole seeds for spouting, dried fruits, pulses, nut butters, soya and vegetable products, sea vegetables, drinks and Bioforce herb tinctures. Write to them for a catalogue. You can order by telephone, fax or post. Pure Multi-Nutrients, 6 Victory Place, Crystal Palace, London, SE19 3RW (Telephone 0181 771 4522, Fax 0181 771 4522)

Soya Milk
My favourite brand of soya milk is Bonsoy. It tastes sweet and the carton is not lined with aluminium.

Udo's Choice
A balance of both omega 3 and omega 6 essential fatty acids as well as other important fatty acids such as GLA. Available from good health food stores or by post from the Nutri Centre (see above). Keep refrigerated and do not heat.

Index